Tongue Body Kinematics in Parkinson's Disease

SPEECH PRODUCTION AND PERCEPTION

Edited by Susanne Fuchs and Pascal Perrier

VOLUME 7

Notes on the quality assurance and peer review of this publication:
Prior to publication, the quality of the work published in this series is
double blind reviewed by external referees appointed by the editorship.
The referee is not aware of the author's name when performing the review;
the referees' names are not disclosed.

Tabea Thies

Tongue Body Kinematics in Parkinson's Disease

Effects of Levodopa and Deep Brain Stimulation

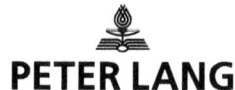

Lausanne • Berlin • Bruxelles • Chennai • New York • Oxford

Bibliographic Information published by the Deutsche Nationalbibliothek
The Deutsche Nationalbibliothek lists this publication in the Deutsche Nationalbibliografie; detailed bibliographic data is available in the internet at http://dnb.d-nb.de.

Library of Congress Cataloging-in-Publication Data
A CIP catalog record for this book has been applied for at the Library of Congress.

Zugl.: Köln, Univ., Diss., 2022

DE-38

ISSN 2191-8651
ISBN 978-3-631-89885-7 (Print)
E-ISBN 978-3-631-89886-4 (E-PDF)
E-ISBN 978-3-631-89887-1 (EPUB)
DOI 10.3726/b20799

© 2023 Peter Lang Group AG, Lausanne
Published by Peter Lang GmbH, Berlin, Deutschland
info@peterlang.com - www.peterlang.com
All rights reserved.

All parts of this publication are protected by copyright. Any utilisation outside the strict limits of the copyright law, without the permission of the publisher, is forbidden and liable to prosecution. This applies in particular to reproductions, translations, microfilming, and storage and processing in electronic retrieval systems.

This publication has been peer reviewed.

www.peterlang.com

Contents

List of Figures 11
List of Tables 13
Acknowledgments 17

1 Introduction 19

2 Parkinson's Disease 23
- 2.1 Pathology 24
  - 2.1.1 Braak Staging 24
  - 2.1.2 Basal Ganglia and the Role of Dopamine 25
- 2.2 Clinical Symptoms and Progression 28
  - 2.2.1 Non-motor Symptoms 28
  - 2.2.2 Motor Symptoms 29
- 2.3 Therapeutic Options 31
  - 2.3.1 Drug Treatment 31
  - 2.3.2 Deep Brain Stimulation 32
- 2.4 Assessing Motor Functions and Treatment Effects 36
  - 2.4.1 Motor Score 36
  - 2.4.2 Calculating the Levodopa and DBS Response 38

3 Speech Production 41
- 3.1 Process of Speech Production 41
- 3.2 Articulatory Speech Movements 43
  - 3.2.1 Articulatory Phonology 43
  - 3.2.2 Dynamical Systems 46
  - 3.2.3 Articulatory Landmarks 48
  - 3.2.4 Timing and Phasing 49
- 3.3 Modifications of Articulatory Movements 51

| | | 3.3.1 Compensation Strategies... | 53 |
| | | 3.3.2 Prominence Marking.. | 55 |

4 Speech in Parkinson's Disease 63

	4.1	Hypokinetic Dysarthria...	63
		4.1.1 Intelligibility and Naturalness.............................	63
		4.1.2 Respiratory-Phonatory Control...........................	65
		4.1.3 Articulation...	67
		4.1.4 Underlying Kinematics.....................................	70
		4.1.5 Prosodic Characteristics	73
		4.1.6 Speech Rate and Fluency	76
	4.2	Development of Speech Deficits	77
	4.3	Treatment Effects on Speech	79
		4.3.1 Effects of Levodopa	79
		4.3.2 Effects of Deep Brain Stimulation	82
		4.3.3 Levodopa vs DBS	89
	4.4	Research Questions	90

5 Methods... 93

	5.1	Objectives	93
	5.2	Participants...	93
	5.3	Data Elicitation	95
		5.3.1 Preoperative Assessment..................................	97
		5.3.2 Postoperative Assessment................................	97
	5.4	Speech Recordings...	99
		5.4.1 Set-up...	99
		5.4.2 Speech Task and Speech Material	100
	5.5	Speech Data Processing	104
		5.5.1 Annotation	105
		5.5.2 Measurements...	107
	5.6	Statistical Analysis...	112

6 Results: Disease Effect 115
6.1 General Assessment 115
6.2 Speech Assessment 116
6.2.1 Speech Ratings 118
6.2.2 Acoustics 118
6.2.3 Articulation 120
6.3 Interim Conclusion 126

7 Results: Levodopa Effect 129
7.1 Motor Assessment 129
7.2 Speech Assessment 130
7.2.1 Speech Ratings 130
7.2.2 Acoustics 131
7.2.3 Articulation 133
7.3 Correlations 136
7.4 Interim Conclusion 137

8 Results: DBS Effect 139
8.1 Motor Assessment 139
8.2 Speech Assessment 140
8.2.1 Speech Ratings 140
8.2.2 Acoustics 141
8.2.3 Articulation 142
8.3 Correlations 145
8.4 Interim Conclusion 146

9 Results: Levodopa vs STN-DBS 147
9.1 Motor Assessment 147
9.2 Speech Assessment 147
9.2.1 Speech Ratings 147

    9.2.2 Acoustics 148
    9.2.3 Articulation 149
  9.3 Interim Conclusion 150

10 Results: Electrode Effect 153
  10.1 General Assessment 153
  10.2 Speech Assessment 155
    10.2.1 Speech Ratings 155
    10.2.2 Acoustics 155
    10.2.3 Articulation 156
    10.2.4 Correlation 158
  10.3 Interim Conclusion 159

11 Discussion 161
  11.1 Disease Effect 161
  11.2 Levodopa Effect 164
  11.3 DBS Effect 165
  11.4 Electrode Effect 167
  11.5 Prominence Marking 169
  11.6 Compensation Strategies 171
  11.7 Variation 173
  11.8 Clinical Implications 175
  11.9 Limitations 176

12 Conclusion 179

Appendix 181
  A.1 Stimulation Parameters 181
  A.2 Neuropsychological Assessment 182

A.3 Characteristics of Dysarthria 184
A.4 Results Motor Assessment 185
A.5 Levodopa Equivalent Daily Doses 188

References 189

List of Figures

Figure 2.1: Neural structures involved in motor control. 27
Figure 2.2: Clinical symptoms and progression of Parkinson's disease 29
Figure 2.3: Schematized DBS electrode. 34
Figure 3.1: Speech process from production to perception. 41
Figure 3.2: Dimensions of tract variables. 45
Figure 3.3: Schematized articulatory movement and relevant landmarks. 48
Figure 3.4: Acoustic-articulatory relationship in a CV syllable. 50
Figure 3.5: Coupling modes in CV and CCV syllables. 50
Figure 3.6: Articulatory modification possibilities. 52
Figure 3.7: Degrees of prosodic prominence. 57
Figure 3.8: Prosodic adjustments on the acoustic level. 58
Figure 3.9: Prosodic adjustments on the articulatory level. 61
Figure 5.1: Location of implanted DBS electrodes. 98
Figure 5.2: Target words. 101
Figure 5.3: Question-answer-scenario for data collection. 102
Figure 5.4: Annotation of articulatory landmarks. 105
Figure 5.5: Examples of different velocity trajectories. 107
Figure 5.6: Acoustic waveform and tongue movement trajectories. ..108
Figure 5.7: Coordination of articulatory movements and acoustic segments. 110
Figure 5.8: Screenshot from SoSci Survey. 111
Figure 6.1: Acoustic vowel duration comparing healthy control speakers and speakers with PD. 119
Figure 6.2: Vowel space area in healthy controls and speakers with PD. 121
Figure 6.3: Tongue body movement comparing healthy control speakers and speakers with PD. 122
Figure 7.1: Levodopa effect on motor functions. 130
Figure 7.2: Speaker-specific changes of acoustic vowel durations after levodopa intake. 132
Figure 7.3: Prosodic adjustments within the acoustic vowel space in med-OFF and med-ON condition. 133
Figure 7.4: Characteristics of tongue body movements after levodopa intake. 134
Figure 8.1: DBS effect on motor functions. 140

Figure 8.2: Speaker-specific changes of acoustic vowel durations under DBS. 142
Figure 8.3: Characteristics of tongue body movements under DBS. ... 143
Figure 9.1: Changes in acoustic vowel duration comparing both treatments. 148
Figure 9.2: Changes of tongue body movements comparing both treatments. 150
Figure 10.1: Motor functions per patient in each OFF condition. 154
Figure 10.2: Changes of tongue body movements comparing both OFF conditions. 157
Figure 10.3: Correlation between motor functions and time passed between assessments. 158
Figure 11.1: Schematized treatment effects on tongue body movements. 164

List of Tables

Table 2.1:	Braak stages.	25
Table 3.1:	Dimensions of tract variables.	45
Table 4.1:	Speech subtypes in Parkinson's disease.	78
Table 5.1:	Demographics of participants.	94
Table 5.2:	Procedure preoperative recording sessions.	97
Table 5.3:	Procedure postoperative recording sessions.	98
Table 5.4:	Examples of question-answer-scenarios.	103
Table 6.1:	Clinical scores of participants.	117
Table 6.2:	Values of the vowel articulation index in the control group and the PD group.	120
Table 6.3:	Movement profile and phases in healthy control speakers and speakers with PD.	124
Table 7.1:	Acoustic vowel durations in med-OFF and med-ON condition.	131
Table 7.2:	Movement profile and phases in med-OFF and med-ON condition.	135
Table 8.1:	Acoustic vowel durations in DBS-OFF and DBS-ON condition.	141
Table 8.2:	Movement profile and phases in DBS-OFF and DBS-ON condition.	144
Table 10.1:	Acoustic vowel durations in med-OFF and DBS-OFF condition.	156
Table 10.2:	Movement profile and phases in med-OFF and DBS-OFF condition.	157
Table A.1:	Individual stimulation settings.	181
Table A.2:	Assessments scores of Beck-Depression-Inventory-II.	182
Table A.3:	Test results of the PANDA.	183
Table A.4:	Results of the Mini-Mental State Examination.	183
Table A.5:	Composition of dysarthric symptoms per individual with PD.	184
Table A.6:	Motor scores of healthy control participants.	185
Table A.7:	Motor scores in med-OFF condition.	186
Table A.8:	Motor scores in med-ON condition.	186
Table A.9:	Motor scores in DBS-OFF condition.	187
Table A.10:	Motor scores in DBS-ON condition.	187
Table A.11:	Amount of PD drugs per patient.	188

Abstract

Introduction: Parkinson's disease (PD) affects not only gross motor but also speech motor control. Speakers with PD exhibit slower, smaller and imprecise articulatory movements, resulting in an overall reduced vowel space and less intelligible speech (Duffy, 2019). The reduced vowel space is related to overall disease severity, but it can increase with dopaminergic treatment (Thies et al., 2021). Standard treatment options are levodopa intake or – in later disease stages – deep brain stimulation (DBS). For DBS, two electrodes are implanted in specific brain areas, such as the nucleus subthalamicus (STN). The effect of both treatments on motor speech is under debate. The goal of this thesis is to investigate the effect of PD, levodopa, and STN-DBS on vocalic tongue movements in the same group of speakers with PD.

Methods: 13 patients which had been diagnosed with PD eight years prior to study inclusion and 13 age- and sex-matched healthy controls participated in the speech production task. All participants were recorded with an electromagnetic articulograph (AG 501) producing ten different target words embedded in carrier sentences in three different controlled focus conditions. Target words were disyllabic girl names ($C_1V_1.C_2V_2$-structure). The vowel V1 was one of the following five German vowels: /i, e, a, o, u/. Acoustic vowel durations of V1, the vowel articulation index, underlying tongue body kinematics (durations, amplitudes, peak velocities), and timing patterns of vocalic movements were calculated.

While healthy speakers were recorded once, speakers with PD were recorded in four different treatment conditions: Before the implantation of DBS electrodes in medication-OFF (without levodopa) and medication-ON condition (with a standardized dose of soluble levodopa), and nine months after DBS implantation without any medication in DBS-OFF (deactivated DBS) and DBS-ON condition (activated DBS). Speech parameters were compared across the groups and treatment conditions. Moreover, 165 naive listeners rated the perceived intelligibility and naturalness of all participants' utterances. In addition, the motor abilities of all participants were assessed in accordance with part III of the Unified Parkinson's Disease Scale.

Results: The results reveal that motor functions and intelligibility improve in consequence of both treatments. While motor functions change in the same direction, results on speech parameters are variable and effects less clear. Nevertheless, both treatments lead to tongue body movements being modulated in time and space. Following levodopa intake, tongue body movements become longer and larger in most of the patients, while movements become shorter and smaller under DBS. Longer and larger movements indicate hyper-articulation, while shorter and smaller movements indicate hypo-articulation. When comparing preoperative and postoperative movements, without the influence of any treatment, tongue body movements tend to be smaller and slower. Timing patterns remain stable across all conditions .

In comparison to the speech of healthy controls, the speech of speakers with PD is slowed down, less intelligible and less natural. According to the naive listeners ratings, intelligibility is lower in speakers with PD that have smaller acoustic vowel spaces and pronounced axial motor impairment.

Conclusion: Both levodopa and activated DBS improve speech motor performance and intelligibility in this sample of patients with PD. Under levodopa, tongue body movements are more agile and precise (longer and larger). With activated DBS, movement durations and amplitudes decrease indicating a lower speech effort. The data further suggests that the mere presence of DBS electrodes worsens the patients' speech ability, as postoperative movement patterns were slower and smaller compared with preoperative patterns. However, the speech system of speakers with PD is flexible enough to control speech parameters in time and space to maintain goal-directed speech production under treatment.

Keywords: Parkinson's disease, articulation, speech kinematics, levodopa, deep brain stimulation

Acknowledgments

I am not a woman of many words. And those that I did have to say I left on the next pages. Nevertheless, I would like to express my deepest gratitude to those people without whom this work would not have become what it is now. Therefore, I would like to thank especially the following people for supporting me:

- **Participants:** For your time and participation in my study.
- **Doris Mücke:** For years of mentorship, giving me advice and support whenever it was needed.
- **Michael T. Barbe:** For introducing me to the neurological world and for entrusting me with your patients.
- **Antje Mefferd:** For your support and for helping me gain a new perspective on articulatory data.
- **Theo Klinker:** For your technical support and the many hours you spent with me on the EMA recordings.
- **Richard Dano:** For teaching me the procedure of the UPDRS motor assessment and its evaluation.
- **Jane Mertens & Gilly Shapira-Mertens:** For your creativity and the artistic realization of the stimuli.
- **Stefan Baumann:** For lending me your voice for the questions asked in the question-answer-scenario.
- **Lukas Henne:** For implementing the question-answer-scenario in a game-like application and extracting my data.
- **Janine Schreen & Kyra Kashigin & Sophie Berlet:** For the time and nerves you put into labeling parts of the data.
- **Hannah Jergas:** For your blinded ratings of the UPDRS and for extracting and visualizing the electrode positions.
- **Bodo Winter & Maximilian Hörl:** For your advice regarding the statistical analysis.
- **Simon Roessig:** For the technical support in R and statistical advice.
- **Christine Röhr:** For your advice regarding the perception experiment and for involving me so early in research.

- **Nuria Geerts & Jonathan Hannemann & Michelle Kühn:** For helping me during the assessments and recordings.
- **Anne Hermes:** For your support and feedback as well as for involving me so early in research.
- **Eduardo Möking:** For being the only one to proofread this dissertation in its entirety before I handed in.

In addition, I have received financial support, which made the realization of the project possible. In the first place, the a.r.t.e.s. Graduate School for the Humanities Cologne should be mentioned here, which, together with the Mercator Foundation, awarded me with a four-year scholarship. In addition, this PhD project was associated with the project A04 "Dynamic modelling of prosodic prominence" as part of the CRC 1252 "Prominence in Language" (German Research Foundation, Project-ID 281511265) at the University of Cologne. The Thiemann Foundation's Visitor Program allowed me to visit Antje Mefferd's lab in Nashville, TN (USA), which had a significant impact on the analysis of the data. Last but not least, I would like to thank the Brain Modulation and Speech Motor Control Team in Cologne for years of support.

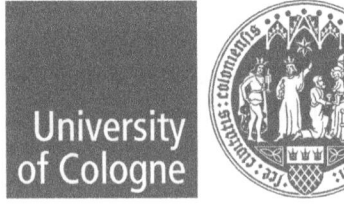

This doctoral dissertation was accepted by the Faculty of Arts and Humanities of the University of Cologne in 2022.

1 Introduction

Speech production requires the ability to coordinate articulatory movements of the speech motor system to produce different consonant and vowel patterns on the textual tier and to adjust them depending on rather complex demands of the communication process. But what happens if this ability is affected by reduced motor skills as it is the consequence of Parkinson's disease? This dissertation aims to investigate the speech production of patients with Parkinson's disease in different medical treatment conditions, and by varying prosodic contexts of the speech material different speech demands are placed on the speech motor system, to better describe and understand the speech system in Parkinson's disease.

Parkinson's disease (PD) is one of the most common movement disorders, whose prevalence increases with age (Hoehn, 1992). Especially in an aging population, the number of patients will increase significantly by 50 % until 2030 (Dorsey et al., 2007). This does not only lead to a growing number of patients with PD but moreover to a growing demand for satisfactory treatment options. All motor and non-motor symptoms that go along with PD are well investigated and characterized with effective therapy options being available to improve motor functions. However, relative to gross motor impairments, speech motor impairments due to PD are less understood.

Since Parkinson's disease is a movement disorder, it affects not only gross motor control, such as the coordination of limbs, but also gross motor performance in terms of smaller, slower, and less extended motions of the limbs. However, not much is known about the effect of PD on the speech motor system, such as tongue and lip movements. It is particularly interesting to look at the speech motor system in detail, which does not only provide insights into underlying movement patterns of the articulators, it also increases the understanding of deviations of the speech system associated with dysarthric speech. This helps to improve the management of the disease with regard to speech therapy, as it is a common goal of speech kinematic studies on dysarthric speech to identify the speech motor impairments that negatively impact the speech function. Although effective behavioral speech interventions exist, there is little guidance on therapeutic selections. Furthermore, speech therapy is not personalized despite manifestations of speech abnormalities being varied across individuals with PD. The main obstacles preventing a better selection process are insufficient knowledge of how speakers with PD differ with regard to their speech motor impairments, how the different impairment types can be identified and the inability to predict which speech treatment approach is best for each individual patient.

A number of studies have already described characteristics of the speech disorder that develops in the course of PD and that also impacts the patients' quality of life. Generally, the speech disorder in PD exhibits less intelligible and less natural speech caused by reduced modulation of the speech melody and loudness, and a reduced and centralized articulation space. The influence of treatment methods on speech are strikingly diverse as some studies report deterioration, some improvement and some no change.

Another aspect that is missing is a detailed look at vowel production, especially on the kinematic level. For this reason, this dissertation aims to shed light on articulatory tongue body movements and how these change due to the disease itself. Articulatory data are beneficial to describe which processes occur below the acoustic surface and further evoke the perceptual impression. Therefore, the special interest of this study lies on how changes of tongue body movements are reflected in the acoustic speech output and whether they are perceived by listeners.

Furthermore, the effect of two standard treatment methods patients are typically subjected to will be investigated. This dissertation will look into how the speech system reacts to drug treatment with levodopa, on the one hand, and on the other hand, how the speech system reacts to deep brain stimulation (DBS) in the nucleus subthalamicus. The overall goal is to further describe how the speech system in PD can adapt to new circumstances and/or external effects, such as treatment methods. At the same time, the ability to compensate for deficits in the speech motor control system will be focused on.

For these purposes, articulatory and acoustic speech recordings were made by means of electromagnetic articulography to directly track the movements of the primary constrictors, such as lips and tongue, during syllable production and to relate them to the acoustic surface of speech. Healthy control speakers and speakers with PD were recruited for the study. Speakers with PD participated in four different conditions: Before the implantation of DBS electrodes in i) medication-OFF (without levodopa) and ii) medication-ON condition (with a standardized dose of soluble levodopa), and after the implantation of DBS electrodes without any medication in iii) deactivated DBS and iv) activated DBS condition. In this study it was possible, for a first time, to analyze data of the same patients over a period of time from before surgery to after surgery and to explore speech in more detail by using kinematic measures.

In order to record speech production more comprehensively and to gain insight into different performance demands of speech production, a speech task was chosen that evokes not only active adjustments of speech parameters, but also requires a modification of different degrees of speech motor effort. This was achieved by eliciting target words in different focus conditions. A target word in accented position requires more speech effort than a target word in unaccented position, as speakers use several phonetic cues to express prosodic prominence with respect to focus structure.

In order to allow for a comprehensive discussion of the topic, the work is divided into three main parts. The first part provides an overview of the theoretical background (Chapter 2, 3 and 4), the second part describes the methodology of the experiment in further detail (Chapter 5), and the third part refers to the results of the study and their assessment (Chapter 6, 7, 8, and 9). In detail, the book is structured as follows:

Chapter 2 provides detailed information about Parkinson's disease, its pathology and the resulting motor and non-motor symptoms and how motor symptoms can be assessed. Moreover, treatment options, such as drug treatment with levodopa and surgical treatment with deep brain stimulation, are explained.

Chapter 3 explains the general process of speech production and sheds light on the framework within articulatory movements will be analyzed. This chapter also addresses adjustments of speech movement parameters and describes how these are realized as well as for which reasons speech production changes.

Chapter 4 describes the characteristics of the speech disorder caused by Parkinson's disease and outlines the development of speech deficits.

Changes in speech due to treatment medical and surgical options are presented as well.

Chapter 5 refers to the experiment, its methodology and setup, as well as data processing. In this final section of the theoretical part, the overall research questions are formulated.

From chapter 6 to chapter 10 the results are presented in three different comparisons. First, differences between healthy control speakers and speakers with PD will be delineated to highlight the impact of the disease on speech. Secondly, the levodopa effect will be analyzed. The effect of switching the neurostimulation on and off will be presented subsequently. And ultimately, chapters 9 and 10 outline how speech differs from baseline (before DBS implantation) to postoperative status.

The final chapter 11 situates the findings in the current literature landscape and discusses them in the context of it.

2 Parkinson's Disease

Parkinson's disease (PD) is one of the most common neurodegenerative diseases. Its main features are motor symptoms, such as slowness of movements, stiffer muscles, and tremor. As a neurodegenerative disorder, brain structures will gradually be affected, leading to a progressive worsening of symptoms in the course of the disease. The disease develops long before the first motor symptoms become visible. The period without motor symptoms is called prodromal or presymptomatic stage. In this phase, non-motor symptoms, such as constipation, sleep disorder, and olfactory dysfunction are considered characteristic (Kalia & Lang, 2015). Detailed information about the relevant non-motor and motor symptoms is given in the following sections 2.2.2 and 2.2.1.

The prevalence of PD is about 1 % in people over 60 years of age and increases with age (Tysnes & Storstein, 2017; De Lau & Breteler, 2006). As an aging-related disease, the number of patients with PD will double by 2030 in an aging population (Dorsey et al., 2007) and reach a prevalence of nearly 3 % in individuals older than 85 years (De Rijk et al., 2000). Men in particular are at a greater risk of developing PD (Tysnes & Storstein, 2017; Van Den Eeden et al., 2003), as well as people with constipation (Stirpe et al., 2016; Svensson et al., 2016; Noyce et al., 2012; Abbott et al., 2001), olfactory disorder (Haehner et al., 2007), and REM-sleep behavior disorder (Zhou et al., 2018; Skorvanek et al., 2018; Janković et al., 2015). Other risk factors can be a family history of PD, alcohol consumption, and pesticide exposure (Kalia & Lang, 2015; Noyce et al., 2012). Smoking and coffee drinking are said to be protective factors (Belvisi et al., 2020; Noyce et al., 2012).

Idiopathic Parkinson's disease is a clinical and pathological syndrome (Berg et al., 2014; Shulman et al., 2011). For a standard diagnosis clinicians rely on criteria of typical motor symptoms, but also on neuroimaging revealing structural correlates of Parkinson's disease, such as a DaTSCAN. In this procedure, a patient is given a small amount of a radioactive drug that attaches to dopamine receptors in the brain (Gayed et al., 2015; de la Fuente-Fernández, 2012). This allows the density and location of dopaminergic cells to be visualized. In people with Parkinson's syndrome the density and marked areas will typically be reduced. So far, the origin of PD is largely unclear. However, two approaches are commonly discussed within the community and will be presented in the following section 2.1. One is based on altered neural processes in the brain and the other is related to a progressive deposition of the protein alpha-synuclein in the central nervous system.

2.1 Pathology

The main characteristic of PD is considered to be the progressive loss of specific brain cells (dopaminergic neurons) in the mid brain, more concretely in the substantia nigra (Berg et al., 2014). However, another process seems to precede this gradual cell death. Knowing that PD starts before the first motor symptoms appear, it was recognized that the prodromal phase is accompanied by a pathology within the nervous system. A deposition of the protein alpha-synuclein appears to be the reason for the cell death of dopaminergic neurons in the substantia nigra within the mid brain. To illustrate this process, the following section discusses the deposition of alpha-synuclein first and the role of dopamine in PD afterwards.

2.1.1 Braak Staging

Following recent approaches, the idea of an underlying pathological process proposed by Braak and colleagues has been gaining more significance in recent times. But it should be noted that the Braak stages as a possible origin of PD are still under debate (Burke et al., 2008). According to Braak et al., PD begins as a synuclein-pathology in terms of a deposition in neurological structures affecting autonomic, limbic, and motor systems (Braak et al., 2004, 2002). The deposition of the alpha-synuclein protein is a gradual process that extends throughout the brain: Beginning in the lower brain stem, continuing through the mid brain and the fore brain to finally affecting the cortex (Braak et al., 2003). This path through the brain is divided into six stages that may explain phase and severity of the disease (Table 2.1). The pathology evolves from stage to stage, from presymptomatic to symptomatic and finally to clinical manifestations in all dimensions (Braak et al., 2003, 2002).

Table 2.1. Braak stages indicating the affected part of the brain, the symptoms and the respective stage of PD.

Stage	Part of brain	PD Phase	Symptoms
Stage 1	Hind brain: Medulla	presymptomatic	non-motor: autonomic, olfactory
Stage 2	Hind brain: Pons	presymptomatic	non-motor: sleep disorder
Stage 3	Mid brain: Substantia nigra	symptomatic	motor
Stage 4	Fore brain	symptomatic	motor
Stage 5	Neocortex	clinic	motor & emotional disturbances
Stage 6	Neocortex	clinic	motor & cognitive deviant

The presymptomatic phases are characterized by predominant non-motor symptoms, such as olfactory and sleep disturbances. Once the substantia nigra (specifically the pars compacta, cf. Section 2.1.2) is affected, motor symptoms may manifest and become progressively worse in the later stages (Braak et al., 2003, 2002). When cortical areas are affected, motor symptoms deteriorate and non-motor functions, such as emotional and cognitive abnormalities, emerge.

While the trigger for the deposition is unclear, this process begins in extra nigral structures without the involvement of dopaminergic structures. As soon as the alpha-synuclein pathology reaches the substantia nigra pars compacta, dopaminergic structures are affected and the loss of dopaminergic neurons begins (Braak et al., 2005). The consequence of dopaminergic depletion is described in more detail in the next section.

2.1.2 Basal Ganglia and the Role of Dopamine

The substantia nigra is part of the basal ganglia, a conglomerate of different nuclei, situated in the mid brain, which are involved in motor control, emotion, and cognition (Obeso et al., 2014; Afifi, 2003). The brain nuclei that belong to the basal ganglia are i) substantia nigra, ii) globus pallidus, iii) nucleus subthalamicus, iv) nucleus caudate, and v) putamen (Groenewegen, 2003). Models suggest that the control of motor and non-motor functions takes place across three different circuits along so-called '*cortico-striato-thalamo-cortical*' connections. Therefore, the basal ganglia are highly connected to the cortex and the thalamus. For the purpose of this work, only the circuit for motor control between the basal ganglia and the motor cortex will be addressed. The motor cortex is a region in the frontal lobe, whereas the thalamus consists of grey matter in the diencephalon. Both structures are also located in the fore brain.

Within the anatomic structures of the basal ganglia, dopamine functions as a neurotransmitter in the brain transmitting signals between neurons from one nerve cell to another. Dopaminergic signaling starts from the substantia nigra pars compacta (SNc) and projects to many brain areas (Figure 2.1). With regard to motor control, dopamine controls neural activity between the motor cortex, the basal ganglia, and the thalamus for motor planning and initiating and executing voluntary movements (Afifi, 2003). This means that dopamine is involved in voluntary motor control.

Motor activity is controlled and generated by two different pathways within the cortico-striato-thalamo-cortical connections in the brain which have opposing functions (Alexander & Crutcher, 1990). One pathway is responsible for increasing motor activity, the other for decreasing it (Chakravarthy et al., 2010; Afifi, 2003). In both pathways, the basal ganglia receive a motor-related input signal from the motor cortex and send it back to the cortex via the thalamus (Groenewegen, 2003). Within the basal ganglia, the striatum, consisting of the caudate nucleus, the putamen, and the nucleus subthalamicus (STN), receives the input signal from cortical areas. In contrast, the globus pallidus internus (GPi) and the substantia nigra pars reticula (SNr) are the output nuclei of the basal ganglia, which project back to the thalamus (Chakravarthy et al., 2010; Afifi, 2003). Neural information between the striatum and the thalamus can be transmitted either on a direct or indirect pathway. Both consist of a closed system in which information is passed on by neuronal excitation and inhibition. Which one of these two pathways is chosen depends on dopaminergic projection from the SNc to dopamine receptors in the striatum (Chakravarthy et al., 2010; Afifi, 2003; Groenewegen, 2003).

Both pathways are depicted in Figure 2.1. The direct pathway is activated if a dopamine receptor D1 in the striatum receives chemical dopaminergic messages from the SNc (Gerfen & Wilson, 1996). This dopaminergic projection modulates the striatal activity by inhibiting the activity in the GPi which further disinhibits the thalamus (Pollack, 2001; Afifi, 2003). This disinhibition of the thalamus leads to increased motor activity. In contrast to the direct pathway, the indirect pathway is activated if dopamine attaches to a D2 receptor (Gerfen & Wilson, 1996). This time the striatum signals a disinhibition of the globus pallidus externus (GPe), which leads to a disinhibition of the STN and further leads to an activation of the GPi. An active indirect pathway inhibits thalamic activity and motor activity decreases (Afifi, 2003; Groenewegen, 2003; Pollack, 2001). An interplay between the indirect and direct pathway usually leads to the execution of a planned movement, triggered by a dopaminergic burst before each movement (Chakravarthy et al., 2010).

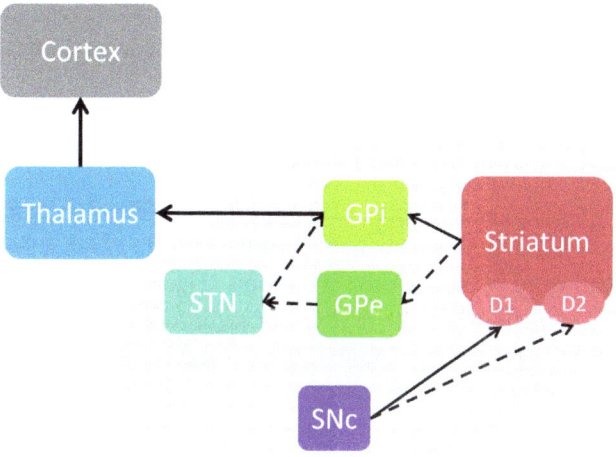

Figure 2.1. Neural structures involved in motor control. The direct pathway is indicated by solid lines, the indirect pathway by dotted lines. Brain nuclei of the basal ganglia are included in the ellipse.

Irregular or altered neural processes in the basal ganglia lead to problems of motor and non-motor functions. Especially the loop between GPe and STN inside the basal ganglia plays an important role, as it supports exploratory behavior (Sridharan et al., 2006). With its excitatory and inhibitory activation possibilities, this neural system produces complex spiking activity (Chakravarthy et al., 2010; Brown et al., 2001). A loss of this complex activity is linked to the pathophysiology of diseases, such as Parkinson's disease (Hasbi et al., 2011; Chakravarthy et al., 2010).

A characteristic of Parkinson's disease is a progressive loss of dopaminergic neurons in the SNc followed by a reduced dopamine concentration in the striatum (Weicker et al., 2001). This in turn leads to striatal disinhibition, which enhances the activity of the indirect pathway and reduces the activity of the direct pathway at the same time. As a result, the inhibition of the thalamus is increased, thereby reducing motor activity (Kern & Kumar, 2007; Weicker et al., 2001).

To summarize, as soon as the alpha-synuclein pathology reaches the substantia nigra, dopaminergic structures are affected and generate a dysregulation of circuits in the basal ganglia, which are inter alia responsible for motor execution and non-motor functions (Chakravarthy et al., 2010; Afifi, 2003). Following on from this, the next chapter covers the description of motor as well as non-motor symptoms of PD.

2.2 Clinical Symptoms and Progression

The pathophysiological correlate of PD appears 10 to 20 years before diagnosis (Kalia & Lang, 2015). During this time, patients are in a prodromal phase, characterized by non-motor symptoms (Figure 2.2). The diagnosis of PD is usually made when the first motor symptoms appear that can be linked to clinical signs, such as bradykinesia, rigidity, and tremor.

2.2.1 Non-motor Symptoms

As described above, PD most likely starts with non-motor symptoms, such as autonomic and olfactory dysfunction (Haehner et al., 2007), constipation (Stirpe et al., 2016; Svensson et al., 2016; Abbott et al., 2001), or a REM-sleep behavior disorder (RBD) (Zhou et al., 2018; Skorvanek et al., 2018; Janković et al., 2015). Depression is an early non-motor symptom as it seems to be a primary consequence of dopaminergic depletion (Tandberg et al., 1997), affecting one third of patients (Aarsland et al., 2012). In later stages of the disease, pain, orthostatic hypotension (reduced blood pressure), incontinence, and sexual dysfunctions may reduce the patients' quality of life further (Schapira et al., 2017). Moreover, neuropsychiatric symptoms, such as anxiety, fatigue, mild cognitive impairment (MCI) or hallucinations, evolve (Figure 2.2). A strong cognitive decline in the form of dementia occurs in 80 % of patients after 20 years of disease (Hely et al., 2008). To conclude, non-motor symptoms include sensory, vegetative, psychiatric, and cognitive symptoms.

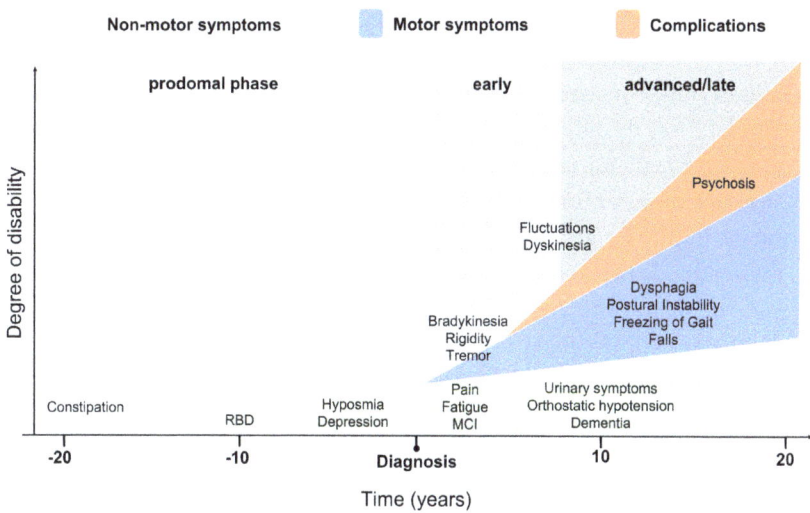

Figure 2.2. Clinical symptoms and progression along a period of 20 years before and 20 years after the diagnosis of PD. Figure is adapted from Kalia and Lang (2015, p. 898).

2.2.2 Motor Symptoms

The loss of about 60 % of dopaminergic cells results in motor manifestations (Obeso et al., 2014; Shulman et al., 2011). Clinically, PD is manifested when at least two cardinal motor symptoms appear. These include bradykinesia, rigidity, and tremor (Deuschl et al., 2016; Fahn, 2003).

Bradykinesia is the cardinal symptom of PD. It refers to difficulties in initiating voluntary movements and slowness of movements. Furthermore, movement amplitude and speed are reduced and decrement over time when patients perform rapid sequential movements (Deuschl et al., 2016; Kalia & Lang, 2015). The symptom of bradykinesia can further be divided into akinesia, referring to initiation disturbances, and hypokinesia, meaning reduced movement amplitudes. Rigidity in the wrist or elbow joint is based on stiffness and an increased muscle tone (Deuschl et al., 2016). A tremor can occur at rest, in a holding position or during activity. The resting tremor is the most common form and occurs with a frequency of 4 to 6 Hz, which is usually visible in the upper and lower limbs, but reduces with activity (Deuschl et al., 2016).

In later stages of the disease, axial symptoms such as postural instability, gait difficulties, dysphagia, and dysarthria appear (Kalia & Lang, 2015). Note that dysphagia (swallowing difficulties) can be an early symptom, but usually no attention is paid to it. Patients do not report swallowing problems until they are more severe, which only then attract the attention of physicians. More details on speech effects are described in chapter 4.1. One of the main problems in advanced PD concerns gait difficulties, such as small-step gait, freezing of gait or falls (Frenklach et al., 2009), which affect 80 % of patients (Hely et al., 2005).

PD symptoms are very heterogeneous across patients. However, clinical subtypes can be defined, depending on the main motor symptoms or the disease onset (Kalia & Lang, 2015; Eggers et al., 2011; Selikhova et al., 2009; Lewis et al., 2005). Patients with a disease onset before the age of 50 are considered early-onset (Schrag & Schott, 2006), while those with an onset above the age of 70 are considered late-onset PD patients (Mehanna et al., 2014; Gibb & Lees, 1988). Within the first five years after being diagnosed with PD, patients are considered as early-stage patients (Kalia & Lang, 2015; Schüpbach et al., 2007). 10 years after diagnosis they are considered to be in an advanced stage (Figure 2.2).

Based on motor symptoms it is possible to additionally differentiate clinical subtypes, such as tremor-dominant and non-tremor dominant PD. Patients with tremor-dominant PD mainly show a (resting) tremor and in general a slower disease progression (Jankovic et al., 1990). The non-tremor-dominant type can further be divided into the akinetic-rigid and the equivalent subtype. While patients with predominantly akinetic-rigid symptoms are assigned to the akinetic-rigid type, patients who have all main symptoms, such as tremor, rigidity, and akinesia, belong to the equivalent type. Recent approaches further take into account non-motor symptoms and disease progression for subtyping (Lawton et al., 2018; Berg et al., 2014).

2.3 Therapeutic Options

Therapy options in Parkinson's disease are only aimed at symptoms, but usually do not prevent the progress of PD (Kalia & Lang, 2015). However, depending on the disease progression, several treatment options exist. In the initial stage drug therapy is the first option, while in advanced stages of the disease either a pump-delivered therapy or deep brain stimulation are further treatment options. For this study, only the treatment of motor symptoms with medication and deep brain stimulation are relevant. Therefore the following sections will focus on these two treatments exclusively. Their aim is to improve activity in dopaminergic circuits to increase motor functions.

2.3.1 Drug Treatment

In the initial stage, patients with PD are treated with drugs aiming to replace the loss of dopamine, such as levodopa or dopamine agonists, to improve motor functions. Dopamine replacement therapy is used since 1960 (Fahn, 2003; Katzenschlager & Lees, 2002). As an active dopamine precursor, levodopa is transformed into dopamine and raises the dopamine concentration in the brain. Dopamine agonists on the other hand directly stimulate the dopamine receptors (Kalia & Lang, 2015; Katzenschlager & Lees, 2002). To improve tremor control, anticholinergic drugs are applied. The composition of the individual drug components varies from patient to patient. The daily dose of anti-parkinsonism drugs taken by a patient can be calculated by using a tool developed by Tomlinson et al. (2010). It allows different drug regimens to be reported in a consistent and comparable manner across patients.

In general, levodopa has a positive effect on motor symptoms and may slow down disease progression (Parkinson Study Group, 2004). However, axial symptoms, often appearing later in the course of the disease, such as gait, postural stability or speech disorder (dysarthria), seem to be less responsive to levodopa treatment compared to other motor symptoms and are considered as treatment-resistant (Kalia & Lang, 2015; Rascol et al., 2003).

As the disease progresses, drug therapy becomes less effective and motor complications appear. Many patients experience the *end-of-dose* or *wearing-off phenomenon*, as levodopa dosages have an increasingly short effect and become less sufficient over time. As a result, the number of drug intakes and regular doses per day increase, meaning that the more advanced the degeneration, the smaller the therapeutic window. It is possible that high levodopa dosages cause involuntary muscle movements of the upper and/or lower extremities, so-called *levodopa-induced dyskinesia*. They are evoked by an enhanced activity in the direct pathway based on more dopamine in the brain than necessary. In this case, a hypokinesia turns into a hyperkinesia caused by a high amount of doperminergic neural activity.

Other long-term complications are motor and non-motor fluctuations (Kalia & Lang, 2015). Fluctuating patients alter between a state of good motor control and periods of reduced motor functions with more severe symptoms (Kalia & Lang, 2015). Changes between a good and a bad motor state may be abrupt and are often not predictable. Other side effects of PD medication are impulse control disorders, which affect 15 % of patients (Weintraub et al., 2010). The prevalence is much higher in combination with dopaminergic agonists. Impulse control disorders include behavioral symptoms, e.g. gambling, compulsive shopping, and hypersexuality. Drug-induced psychosis is rare but can also appear.

Patients suffering from tremor-dominant PD with medication-resistant tremor as well as patients with motor fluctuations, levodopa-induced dyskinesia, and therapy-refractory PD are candidates for the more invasive treatment method of a deep brain stimulation (Lozano et al., 2019; Commissioning Board, 2013; Limousin & Martinez-Torres, 2008), which will be explained in the following section.

2.3.2 Deep Brain Stimulation

Deep brain stimulation (DBS) is an invasive neurosurgical treatment option for movement disorders, such as essential tremor, dystonia, and Parkinson's disease. DBS was approved for treating a more broad range of syndromes by the Food and Drug Administration (FDA) in the 1990s (Benabid, 2003). In this procedure, electrodes, usually one per hemisphere, are surgically implanted in specific areas of the patients' brain, which then stimulate brain nuclei with electrical pulses. Three different brain nuclei can function as target regions for the stimulation in PD: GPi in the pallidum, nucleus ventralis intermedius (VIM) in the thalamus and the STN. The aim of DBS is to stabilize altered neuronal processes and reduce motor dysfunctions by modulating the activity of the basal ganglia.

However, the mechanism of DBS is not entirely understood yet (Kern & Kumar, 2007). DBS is expected to improve the neural activity in the basal ganglia in patients with PD by stimulating either region around the GPi or the STN (Lozano et al., 2019) to balance the activity across the direct and indirect pathway (cf. Section 2.1.2): *"Surgical interventions targeting the STN and GPi may alleviate Parkinsonism by reducing the excessive inhibitory output of the basal ganglia"* (Kern & Kumar, 2007, p. 239).

Set-up and Electrode Implantation

The DBS hardware consists of a pulse generator, cables, and electrodes. Micro-electrodes in the brain are connected via a cable to a pulse generator, which is typically implanted under the skin around the chest (Kern & Kumar, 2007). The pulse generator provides a continuous electrical stimulation of the target area around the implanted electrodes. Electrodes can be implanted either unilaterally in only one hemisphere, or bilaterally in both hemispheres. Each electrode contains four contact levels from which stimulation can be spread into brain structures (Figure 2.3). The latest electrode variants allow circular stimulation in a so-called ring-mode on the lowest and highest contact levels and segmented stimulation with three contacts per level in the two middle ones (Frey et al., 2022). The segmented contacts allow the activation of stimulation either on one third, two thirds or even on the whole ring. This allows for more targeted stimulation of specific brain structures.

The stimulation settings can be changed according to frequency (Hz), pulse width (μs), voltage (V), amplitude (mA), and active stimulating contacts (Benabid, 2003; Ramasubbu et al., 2018). Clinical effects of DBS can often be seen within seconds, but stimulation parameters need to be adjusted in the course of the disease to maximize the treatment effect and to reduce side effects (Kern & Kumar, 2007; Ramasubbu et al., 2018).

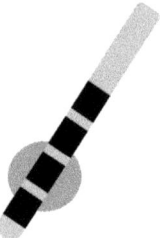

Figure 2.3. Schematized DBS electrode with four contacts from which stimulation can be activated. The gray circle indicates active stimulation of the second contact.

Not every patient is suitable for DBS. Therefore, patients who are eligible for this procedure are examined and determined by a multidisciplinary team consisting of neurologists, neurosurgeons, neuropsychologists, and psychiatrists (Lozano et al., 2019; Kern & Kumar, 2007). While neurologists are involved in making the final diagnosis, determining the dopa-responsiveness of symptoms (see Section 2.4.2 on levodopa challenge test) and deciding which clinical symptoms should be treated with the DBS, neurosurgeons assess the surgery risk and perform the surgery. Furthermore, neuropsychologists perform cognitive testing (Kern & Kumar, 2007) and psychiatrists speak extensively with patients to identify psychiatric problems which could interfere with a DBS indication. Contraindications for DBS are anxiety, depression, psychosis, mania, hallucinations or a pronounced impulse control disorder.

Target Regions and Treatment Effects

If a patient is considered to be suitable for DBS implantation, the target for stimulation needs to be determined. Electrode implantation in the VIM is mostly used for patients with essential tremor as it improves nearly 80 % of the action tremor (Iorio-Morin et al., 2020). In contrast, VIM-DBS is no longer recommend as a treatment for PD (Kumar et al., 1999; Krack et al., 1997), since despite the tremor it does not affect other PD symptoms. In a few cases, VIM-DBS is implanted in elderly patients with tremor-dominant PD without further PD symptoms (Lind et al., 2008).

Popular areas for electrode implantation in PD are the sensimotor parts of the GPi and the STN (Iorio-Morin et al., 2020; Lozano et al., 2019; Limousin & Martinez-Torres, 2008; Krack et al., 2001). Both targets sufficiently improve motor functions, decrease the periods of poor mobility and therefore improve activities of daily living (Follett et al., 2010; Moro et al., 2010; Vitek, 2002; Kumar et al., 1998). Depending on the indication, either one nucleus is targeted or the other, as risks and advantages vary.

GPi stimulation leads to improved depression, bradykinesia, less tremor, and suppresses dyskinesia (Moro et al., 2010; Follett et al., 2010). However, the total daily dose of PD medication often remains unchanged after surgery (Moro et al., 2010). In contrast to GPi-DBS, patients with STN-DBS can reduce the medication dosages by at least 35 % (Liang et al., 2006; Rodriguez-Oroz et al., 2005; Kumar et al., 1998), sometimes by up to 50 % (Benabid, 2003). Additionally, motor symptoms such as bradykinesia, tremor, and rigidity can be reduced, dyskinesia improved and periods of reduced motor functions shortened (Zhang et al., 2006; Rodriguez-Oroz et al., 2005). Side effects of STN stimulation can be changes in mood and behavior, such as a worsening of preexisting depressive symptoms (Lozano et al., 2019; Follett et al., 2010; Rodriguez-Oroz et al., 2005; Vitek, 2002). A general disadvantage is that especially psychiatric symptoms can appear or already existing symptoms worsen. However, a recent study reports that sleep, fatigue, mood, and cognition can also improve after STN-DBS and GPi-DBS (Dafsari et al., 2020).

Besides the improved quality of life due to DBS, the disease still progresses and axial symptoms, which develop and enhance in the later stages of the disease, are considered stimulation-refractory. Therefore, gait, postural instability as well as speech are less sensitive to DBS (Lozano et al., 2019; Benabid, 2003), and freezing of gait in particular rarely improves with DBS (Pötter-Nerger & Volkmann, 2013). In addition, some patients may suffer from stimulation induced speech problems (Kumar et al., 1998). However, another study suggests that DBS can be a better treatment for PD compared to drug treatment (Schüpbach et al., 2007).

Time from Implantation to Symptom Improvement

One aspect to be mentioned in the context of DBS and symptom improvement is the so-called *micro lesion effect*. The micro lesion effect refers to the impact of electrode implantation on motor symptoms immediately after surgery but before the activation of electrical stimulation (Mestre et al., 2016; Cersosimo et al., 2009; Maltête et al., 2008; Kumar et al., 1998). It appears that the mere presence of electrodes in the brain has a positive effect on the motor system. Patients with bradykinesa have shown improved motor functions in the form of faster boxing movements upon electrode implantation (Singh et al., 2012). It is assumed that the improvement is mainly caused by local edema around the area of implanted electrodes but the reason remains unclear.

Aside from that, there is a correlation between the micro lesion effect and the DBS effect, as the degree of motor improvement caused my micro lesion predicts the effect DBS will have on motor functions (Lange et al., 2022; Wang et al., 2017; Tykocki et al., 2013; Maltête et al., 2008): Higher motor improvement based on micro lesion indicates an even greater effect of activated DBS. Most of the patients experience this phenomenon, provided that electrodes are implanted in the right position. However, this improvement is temporary and last about at least 24 to 72 hours and up to a maximum of three weeks (Wang et al., 2017; Cersosimo et al., 2009; Limousin & Martinez-Torres, 2008). In addition to the micro lesion effect, the *placebo effect* has shown to improve motor functions in PD as well. It was observed that motor improvement can be triggered by the patients' expectations of the treatment (Keitel et al., 2013; Mercado et al., 2006; de la Fuente-Fernández et al., 2004).

In contrast to the reported short-term effects, it takes some time for the stimulation effect to stabilize in the long-term after activating the stimulation. Usually stimulation parameters need to be adjusted a few times in the period following the activation, but they remain stable after three months, or at six months at the latest, after surgery (Mestre et al., 2016; Castrioto et al., 2013; Kern & Kumar, 2007; Kumar et al., 1998) when microhemorrhages or edema are resolved (Cersosimo et al., 2009).

2.4 Assessing Motor Functions and Treatment Effects

2.4.1 Motor Score

To monitor disease progression and severity, treatment effects, but also side effects, a tool was developed in 1987 called the *Unified Parkinson's Disease*

Rating Scale (UPDRS; Fahn, Elton, & Committee, 1987). The original scale consists of six parts focusing on relevant non-motor and motor symptoms. Part I to part IV are specific parts of the UPDRS, while part V and VI include previously established rating scales for the assessment of PD.

- **Part I:** 4 items assessing mentation, behavior, and mood.
- **Part II:** 13 items assessing activities of daily living.
- **Part III:** 14 items examining motor functions.
- **Part IV:** 11 items assessing therapy complications in the past week, such as dyskinesia or fluctuations.
- **Part V:** Classification of the stage of PD according to a modified Hoehn and Yahr Scale (Goetz et al., 2004).
- **Part VI:** Classification of activities of daily living according to the scale of Schwab and England (Schwab, 1969).

Parts I to III are scored on a 0 to 4 scale where higher scores indicate a greater impairment (0 = normal, 4 = severely impaired). Part III of the UPDRS is relevant for monitoring the motor functions. Motor examinations include, for example, the evaluation of speech, facial expression, tremor, joint rigidity, gait, and posture, as well as speed and amplitude of arm, hand, finger, and leg movements. The maximal score of part III is 108. Usually a video is recorded during the examination of the motor functions.

After criticizing the UPDRS in 2003, a task force of the Movement Disorder Society (MDS) provided a modified version of the UPDRS in 2007 (Goetz et al., 2007), which was sponsored by the International Parkinson and Movement Disorder Society. The new version, MDS-UPDRS, consists of the following four parts (Goetz et al., 2008):

- **Part I:** 13 items assessing non-motor experiences of daily living.
- **Part II:** 13 items assessing motor experience of daily living.
- **Part III:** 18 items assessing motor examination.
- **Part IV:** 6 items assessing motor complications.

As in the previous version, all items are rated on a 0 to 4 scale, on which 0 indicates 'normal' and 4 'most severe'. The main difference is that detailed instructions are given across all items and disturbances of function are described in the respective category to guarantee uniformity (Goetz et al., 2007). Moreover, the assessment of non-motor symptoms was expanded. And in addition, some parts, such as part I, have been modified, to make it possible to specify who answered the questions; patient, caregiver or both together. It is important to note that a permission is required to use the MDS-UPDRS.

By using values of either of the two UPDRS versions, it is possible to calculate subscores that are related do domain-specific symptoms, such as axial symptoms or rigidity. Depending on the subscore, the values of specific categories are added up. For example, within the UPDRS, items 23 to 26 + item 31 would relate to bradykinesia, item 22 to rigidity, item 20 + item 21 to tremor, item 18 + items 27 to 30 to axial symptoms, items 27 to 30 to postural instability and gait difficulties (cf. Rusz, Cmejla, Růžička, et al., 2013). The UPDRS will be used in this study.

2.4.2 Calculating the Levodopa and DBS Response

The UPDRS is the most widely used scale in clinical practice and in research assessing PD, regardless of whether the old or new version is applied. Using part III of the UPDRS or MDS-UPDRS allows the degree of improvement of the levodopa therapy or DBS to be assessed. For this purpose, motor skills in the OFF status (without treatment) are compared with those in the ON status (with treatment) (Pieterman et al., 2018).

The so-called *levodopa challenge test* (Pieterman et al., 2018) examines the effect of a supra-maximal levodopa dosage on motor functions. The motor performances of patients with PD are thereby evaluated in two conditions:

- **Medication-OFF condition:** after 12 hours of PD medication cessation
- **Medication-ON condition:** with a predetermined dose of 200 - 300 mg of soluble levodopa (100/25 mg levodopa/carbidopa tablets)

The scores that both conditions achieve according to part III of the UPDRS are then compared in order to determine the influence levodopa has had on the patients' motor functions. For comparison, either the absolute change $(OFF-ON)$ or the percentage change $((OFF-ON)/OFF*100)$ can be reported. As Pieterman et al. (2018) suggest, the absolute change should be reported rather than the more commonly used percentage change, as the former correlates with disease duration, levodopa intake duration, and the OFF motor score.

The levodopa response indicates the motor improvement from medication-OFF to medication-ON condition, which is predictive of the motor outcome after (STN-)DBS (Pahwa et al., 2006; Charles et al., 2002; Welter et al., 2002). Therefore, the levodopa challenge test is also performed before a possible DBS implantation. To justify electrode implantation, a minimum of 40 % improvement should be reached (Commissioning Board, 2013).

The test can also be performed to capture treatment effects on motor symptoms after DBS implantation, in this case as a *DBS challenge test* comparing DBS-OFF condition and DBS-ON condition by switching the stimulation OFF and ON.

3 Speech Production

3.1 Process of Speech Production

Speaking, or the production of meaningful sounds, is the basis of oral communication with the purpose of exchanging ideas, feelings, information, and much more among interlocutors (Löfqvist, 2010). Within those interactions, speech connects the speaker and the listener, as the speaker produces utterances that the listener receives and understands (Figure 3.1; Neppert, 1999). Cognitive and motor processes are involved in the production of intended utterances. The speaker has to (i) plan an utterance, (ii) choose the linguistic units, and (iii) initiate the right movements of the respective articulators (Levelt, 1993). Therefore, the speech motor process starts with the planning and ends with the execution of speech movements (Duffy, 2019).

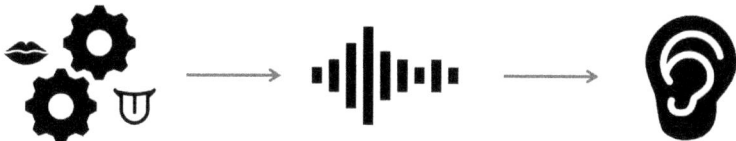

Figure 3.1. Speech process from speakers' articulation via the acoustic signal to the listeners' perception.

The planning process on the cognitive level requires intact cognitive functions, such as attention and working memory (Swets et al., 2013, 2007; Ferreira & Swets, 2002; Levelt & Meyer, 2000). Cognitive-linguistic processes target the discrete linguistic category (phonological form) which needs to be translated into continuous articulatory movement patterns (the phonetic surface) to achieve the intended acoustic output that is perceived by the listener (Harrington & Cassidy, 1999). After planning, the required motor program and relevant motor commands are activated to achieve the intended articulatory and acoustic goals (Löfqvist, 2010). Therefore, the speech motor execution can be understood as a goal-directed process of activating articulatory movements (Goldstein & Fowler, 2003).

The speech motor system is part of the general motor system. Therefore, planning, control, and execution of speech movements is organized in neural structures within the brain (Duffy, 2019). This neural organization of the speech process activates muscles required for speech movements (Löfqvist, 2010). Many neurons and small muscle groups are involved making the neural control process particularly complex. Due to space limitations it will therefore not be covered in greater detail in this work. Moreover, the process of speech motor control is not entirely understood to date. For these reasons, only articulated speech patterns will be focused on in the following.

> *"Speech motor control comprises the adjustment of speed, movement range, and temporal coordination of the muscular activity in a large number of single muscles that contribute to speech breathing, phonation, and articulation."* (Hertrich et al., 2021, p. 337)

The citation above from Hertrich et al. (2021) refers to the variety of speech subsystems and organs in the body that are involved in speech production. Due to the functional circuit of speech production, the respiratory system, the phonatory system, the resonatory system, and the articulatory system are of importance for the production of speech sounds (Duffy, 2019; Ziegler, 2017; Löfqvist, 2010). The speech production process begins with the controlled activation of the expiratory muscles. The air is transported from the lungs to the glottis, which can lead to vocal fold vibration (if desired for the production of voiced sounds). From the vocal folds, the air stream is transported further into the oral and nasal cavity. Depending on the position of the active articulators (jaw, tongue, lips, uvula), specific sounds are produced when the air resonates in the mouth (Neppert, 1999). The sound changes depending on either the position of the articulators or the activity and strength of involved muscles. Note that all subsystems interact with each other: Changes in one speech subsystem can influence the processing in another speech subsystem, as the speech output is the result of the interaction between the source (respiration, phonation) and the filter (vocal tract) (Stevens, 2000). Especially phonation and articulation are dependent on stable breath support, since higher subglottal air pressure influences glottal activity and the amount of acoustic energy that can radiate from the mouth (Ziegler, 2017).

As this dissertation focuses on articulatory properties in speakers with Parkinson's disease, this chapter will mainly concentrate on describing movements of articulators and explains why and how they are modulated.

3.2 Articulatory Speech Movements

The speech subsystem of articulation is related to the movements and positions of active articulators which the acoustic speech output depends on. Active articulators are the lips, the tongue tip, the tongue body, and the jaw. Six distinct parameters influence the characteristics of speech movements. Change in one of these parameters affects all other features as well (Duffy, 2019; Darley et al., 1975):

- **Strength** of muscles required for speech movements.
- **Tone** of speech muscles.
- **Speed** of speech movements.
- **Range** of speech movements.
- **Steadiness** with regard to less variable speed, duration, and range of speech movements.
- **Accuracy** of speech movements as a result of successful regulation and articulatory goal achievement.

Especially speed, range, accuracy, and timing patterns are important when investigating speech movements in Parkinson's disease, which will be further discussed in chapter 4. In the research area of speech production, articulatory events are either observed as raw movements or implemented in the framework of *Articulatory Phonology* and the model of *task dynamics*, which will be explained in the following. Many of the descriptive parameters listed above can also be found in the framework of Articulatory Phonology defining speech movements as described below.

3.2.1 Articulatory Phonology

The framework of Articulatory Phonology makes use of the *task-dynamics model* (AP/TD). This dynamical approach assumes that discrete categories that are presented as phonological forms of speech sounds can be combined with continuous aspects of speech production on the phonetic surface (Saltzman & Munhall, 1989), aiming at *"simultaneously describing phonetics and phonology"* (Iskarous, 2017, p. 2). In AP/TD the basic unit of speech production is an articulatory gesture (Hall, 2010; Browman & Goldstein, 1990). These gestures are on the one hand units of action (phonetic surface), and on the other hand units of contrast (phonological form; Browman & Goldstein, 1992). The gestures' objective is to produce a specific sound and reach a linguistic target, e.g. producing a stop consonant with a bilabial closure (/p/ or /b/).

The aim of reaching a linguistic target classifies speech production as goal-directed actions of different articulators (Goldstein & Fowler, 2003). In the AP/TD framework, gestures are related to coordinated movements within the vocal tract. Each gesture reaches a specific (linguistic) target in order to be audible on the acoustic surface perceived by the listener. Articulatory gestures can be described by so-called tract variables (Browman & Goldstein, 1992).

One tract variable refers to a whole set of articulators that need to be recruited to reach the target within the vocal tract (Browman & Goldstein, 1992; Saltzman & Munhall, 1989). Thus, tract variables do not refer to movements of individual articulators but to groups of articulators that are simultaneously recruited for the production of one gesture. The dimensions in which tract variables can be modulated are presented in Figure 3.2. Gestures of tract variables can be divided into oral, glottal, and velic gestures. While velic and glottal gestures are specified in a single tract variable, oral gestures (lips, tongue tip, and tongue body) are specified pairwise (Browman & Goldstein, 1989). This means that target positions of oral articulatory gestures are described by two descriptors: constriction location and constriction degree. The constriction location (CL) defines the location in the vocal tract to which a gesture moves, and the constriction degree (CD) refers to the level of openness (Goldstein & Fowler, 2003; Browman & Goldstein, 1990; Saltzman & Munhall, 1989). Possible descriptors for the two domains are presented in Table 3.1 (Browman & Goldstein, 1989, p. 209).

Lip gestures, which involve lip and jaw movement, can be modulated in the following dimensions (Figure 3.2): protrusion (LP) and aperture (LA). The jaw is not considered an independent articulator in this framework,

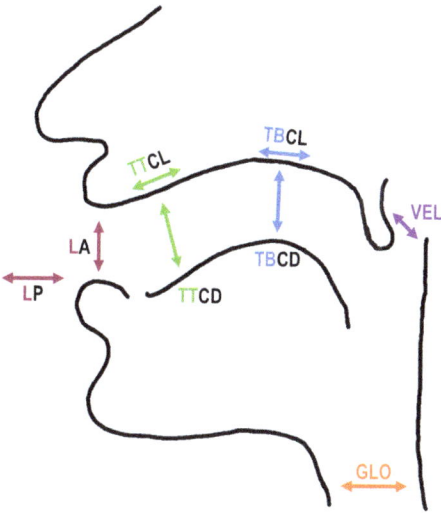

Figure 3.2. Dimensions of tract variables of the lips (L), the tongue tip (TT), the tongue body (TB), the velum (VEL), and the glottis (GLO). Figure adapted from Hall (2010); Browman and Goldstein (1989).

Table 3.1. Dimensions of tract variables divided into constriction location (CL) and constriction degree (CD).

CD descriptors	CL descriptors	
closed	protruded	palatal
critical	labial	velar
narrow	dental	uvular
mid	alveolar	pharyngeal
wide	postalveolar	

as it forms one organ group with the lower lip and another organ group with the tongue, each classified in a single tract variable (Löfqvist, 2010). Tongue movements can be specified for the tongue tip (TT) and tongue body (TB) separately across constriction location (CL) and constriction degree (CD). To give an example: The production of a velar stop consonant requires two oral tract variables to reach a goal. The constriction of the tongue body needs to be located at a 'velar' position with a 'closed' constriction degree between the tongue body and the velum. Tongue movements always form a synergy with the jaw to form a tract variable. Gestures of the glottis (GLO) and the velum (VEL) are characterized in terms of their aperture or closure. The default settings are vibrating focal folds within the glottis and a raised velum. Therefore, indicating voiceless sounds (open vocal folds) and nasalization (lowered velum) requires a *wide* gesture to be introduced as CD in either case.

Movements can be reprogrammed depending on specific requirements during speech production; either due to internal coordination or phonetic and discourse-specific modulations, such as prosodic marking (Löfqvist, 2010; Goldstein & Fowler, 2003; Browman & Goldstein, 1990). As the framework of AP/TD was developed with respect to neurotypical speech production, it is sometimes not adequate to describe impaired speech (Mücke et al., 2022). For example, it has been shown that the tongue body and the jaw do move independently from each other in speakers with PD (Mefferd & Dietrich, 2019). Therefore, the question arises if the jaw should be considered as a separate tract variable. Due to this issue, I will refer to movements instead of phonological gestures from this point onwards with respect to the topic of this dissertation.

3.2.2 Dynamical Systems

The dynamical approach of AP/TD is based on a differential equation, which is the core of dynamical systems. Therefore, the control of speech movements is modeled using the equation of a dynamical system, such as a *mass-spring system*, in order to explain how the system behaves over time (Goldstein & Fowler, 2003; Browman & Goldstein, 1992, 1989; Saltzman & Kelso, 1987; Saltzman, 1986). For the purpose of characterizing speech from an AP/TD perspective, the dynamical system approach describes the motion of tract variables (articulatory events) (Browman & Goldstein, 1992; Saltzman & Kelso, 1987), as the *"primary task in speaking is to control the coordinated movement of sets of articulators"* (Browman & Goldstein, 1990, p. 2). A *damped* mass-spring system based on a second-order differential equation is applied to model coordinated movements that reach a specific spatial target at a certain time (Saltzman & Munhall, 1989). The damping factor is added to the equation to explain that a tract variable reaches a target/equilibrium position and does not constantly oscillate (Iskarous, 2017; Browman & Goldstein, 1990). The following equation 3.1 can be used to describe the evolution of a movement towards a target:

$$ma + bv + k(x - C) = 0 \qquad (3.1)$$

The variable m refers to the mass of an object, a to the acceleration, b to the damping, v to the velocity, k to the stiffness of the spring, x refers to the current position and C to the equilibrium or target position. In a damped mass-spring system the oscillation diminishes with increasing values of b, such that the oscillating object's deflection approaches zero asymptotically, i.e. without reaching it (Mücke, 2018; Iskarous, 2017). This illustrates the movement of an object towards a target position.

For most objects, mass m and damping b are constant, while stiffness k and equilibrium C are variable and the more relevant parameters for modeling speech movements (Mücke, 2018; Browman & Goldstein, 1990). To put the theory into practice, imagine the production of an alveolar closure in the sequence /ata/: x would be the starting position of the tongue with a lowered tongue tip during /a/, and C would be the target position of the tongue tip near the alveolar ridge for /t/. As the characteristics of the tongue itself do not change during the movement, the mass and damping parameters of the tongue remain the same. An important feature of movements in mass-spring systems is that they reach the same target despite different initial positions (Hall, 2010; Browman & Goldstein, 1990). Thus, even when the goal is the same, there are different ways to get there (Perrier & Fuchs, 2015). For example, when comparing the production of the sequences /apa/ and /ipi/, the distance the lower lip has to travel to produce the bilabial plosive depends on its initial position (Mücke, 2018; Turkmani et al., 2007; Macchi, 1988). The distance is longer in /apa/ compared to /ipi/ because the jaw opening and the distance between the lower and upper lip is larger during the production of the open vowel /a/. The phenomenon that speech movements are coordinated with each other in time and space is called coarticulation (Mattingly, 1981). Thus, the AP/TD framework is capable to describe co-articulation and gradient variation that may particularly be generated by impaired speech.

3.2.3 Articulatory Landmarks

From within the AP/TD model, specific landmarks can be defined that describe an articulatory movement (Figure 3.3), such as onset, target, maximal peak velocity, duration and displacement (Mücke, 2018). Onset and target mark the beginning (relative minimum) and the end (relative maximum) of a movement respectively. At both landmarks the velocity of the gestural movement is zero. The time interval between these two landmarks is the movement duration, typically measured in milliseconds. The spatial difference between them is the displacement (or amplitude) of the movement, measured in millimeters. Another parameter is the point in time at which an articulator reaches its maximum speed (peak velocity) while moving to its target, which is measured in millimeters per second or millisecond. From the starting point to the point of peak velocity the articulator accelerates, while it decelerates again before reaching the target. The first interval (onset-to-peak velocity) is the acceleration phase, while the second interval (peak velocity to target) is the deceleration phase of a movement.

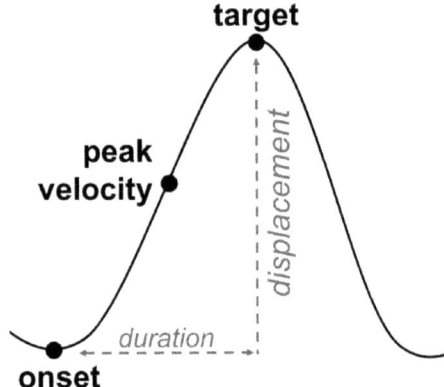

Figure 3.3. Schematized articulatory movement and relevant landmarks that can be specified.

A more abstract but important parameter is the stiffness of a movement. Stiffness describes the time a movement needs to reach its target (or to complete one movement cycle): *"The stiffer the movement, the higher its frequency of oscillation and therefore the less time it takes for one cycle"* (Browman & Goldstein, 1990, p. 6). It refers to the ratio of maximum velocity (mm/s) to the amplitude (mm), as proposed by Munhall, Ostry, and Avraham (1985). Accordingly, stiffness is a spatio-temporal parameter whose values increase as duration decreases.

$$stiffness(k) = \frac{\text{max. velocity}}{\text{amplitude}} \quad (3.2)$$

As already mentioned, these articulatory landmarks can be related to the speech movement features listed above (cf. beginning of Chapter 3.2). Stiffness can be related to the tone of speech muscles, peak velocity to the maximum speed, and amplitude to the range of a movement.

3.2.4 Timing and Phasing

Movements of articulators producing speech sounds are modeled dynamically in time and space (Hall, 2010; Browman & Goldstein, 1992). As speaking is a continuous process of producing different words or sounds that are further composed of several movements (Goldstein et al., 2009), articulatory movements are not realized independently of each other, but are orchestrated with respect to each other in time and space (Browman & Goldstein, 1992, 1990). Thus, articulatory movements while still being present on the articulatory surface, can acoustically mask one another (Hall, 2010). The movements usually overlap only partially because the targets are reached at different times for perceptual recoverability. Thereby, a sound sequence is generated on the acoustic level. Figure 3.4 depicts the underlying articulatory movements for a CV syllable, consisting of one consonant (C) and one vowel (V), and the related acoustic output.

As it can be seen in Figure 3.4, both movements start at the same time, but reach their targets at different moments, which is why a CV sequence is perceived on the acoustic level. The consonantal movement needs less time to achieve the target and is therefore shorter and stiffer. Vocalic movements are less stiff and relatively slow compared to consonantal movements, therefore needing more time to reach their target. While the articulatory targets are reached within their respective acoustic segments, the onset of articulatory movements is timed earlier than the beginning of the acoustic segment or syllable.

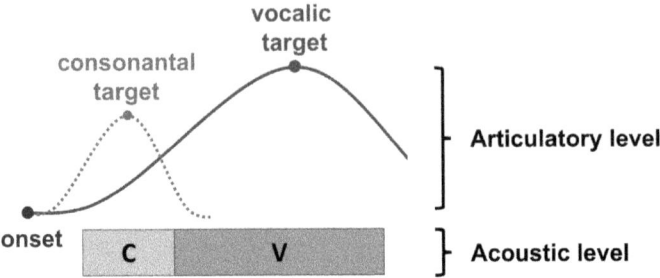

Figure 3.4. Acoustic-articulatory relationship in a CV syllable consisting of one consonant (C) and one vowel (V).

In the theory of AP/TD, articulatory movements are modeled as non-linear oscillators, and can be pictured as working together like stable timing clocks (Iskarous, 2017). The oscillators are coordinated pairwise by specific coupling modes (Goldstein et al., 2009). There are two intrinsic modes that describe the coordination patterns between different articulatory movements: *in-phase* and *anti-phase*. These two timing relations/coupling modes of movements can also be found on the level of syllable structure (Browman & Goldstein, 1988). The examples given are those of a simple CV syllable and a more complex CCV syllable (Figure 3.5).

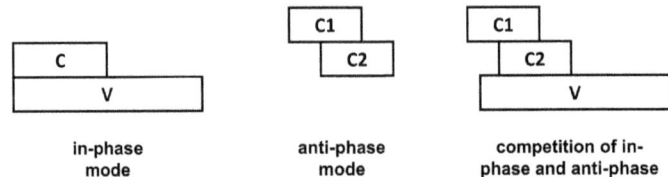

Figure 3.5. Overview over coupling modes in simple CV and complex CCV syllables.

The in-phase coupling mode describes the timing of a consonantal and a vocalic movement within a CV syllable. Both movements start at the same time, as already shown in Figure 3.4. The anti-phase coupling is related to movements that are initiated sequentially. Anti-phase coupling typically occurs in VC syllables, but is also seen in CC sequences. Both coupling modes co-occur in a complex syllable that contains at least two consonants. In a CCV syllable, which forms a complex onset, the timing patterns become competitive because both consonantal movements are coupled in-phase with the vocalic movement, but are coupled in anti-phase with each other for perceptual recoverability (Figure 3.5). Consequently, durational properties, especially of consonants, decrease in more complex syllables (Browman & Goldstein, 1988)[1].

3.3 Modifications of Articulatory Movements

As the AP/TD allows for context-dependent variability (Goldstein & Fowler, 2003), modifications of parameters will result in a different movement trajectory (Mücke, 2018). Intra-movement variation will have consequences on the acoustic outcome (Browman & Goldstein, 1992, 1989). Depending on the contextual requirements, stiffness and target position can vary. Therefore, the length and tension of articulatory movements constantly changes (Hall, 2010, p. 818), but the aim to achieve the desired motor goal or target remains the same (Patri et al., 2015). Different modification strategies exist based on changes in parameters (Mücke, 2018; Mücke et al., 2017).

Changes in articulatory movements include modifications of the target and/ or the stiffness (Figure 3.6). Depending on whether only the target, only the stiffness or both parameters are modified, the movement changes regarding its spatial, temporal or spatio-temporal orientation (Mücke, 2018; Cho, 2006; Beckman et al., 1992). Modifications of only the target height (amplitude) influence the movement amplitude and speed, while modifications of only the stiffness influence movement duration and speed. On the contrary, proportional modifications of both parameters at the same time affect duration and amplitude but not speed. This will be explained in more detail below.

---

1 Read more on the C-Center effect that is present in more complex syllable onsets in some languages (Hermes et al., 2019, 2017; Hoole & Bombien, 2017; Hermes et al., 2013; Marin & Pouplier, 2010; Kühnert et al., 2007).

Modification of Target Height

A modification of the target height leads to a change in the spatial orientation of the movement, as the amplitude either increases or decreases (Figure 3.6, top row). While changes in the spatial dimension also affect the peak velocities, the overall movement duration remains the same in this scenario (Ostry & Munhall, 1985). If the movement amplitude decreases, this leads to a target undershoot and lower peak velocities. Therefore, a target undershoot results in smaller and slower movements. In contrast, a target overshoot is characterized by larger and faster movements, as amplitude and peak velocity increase.

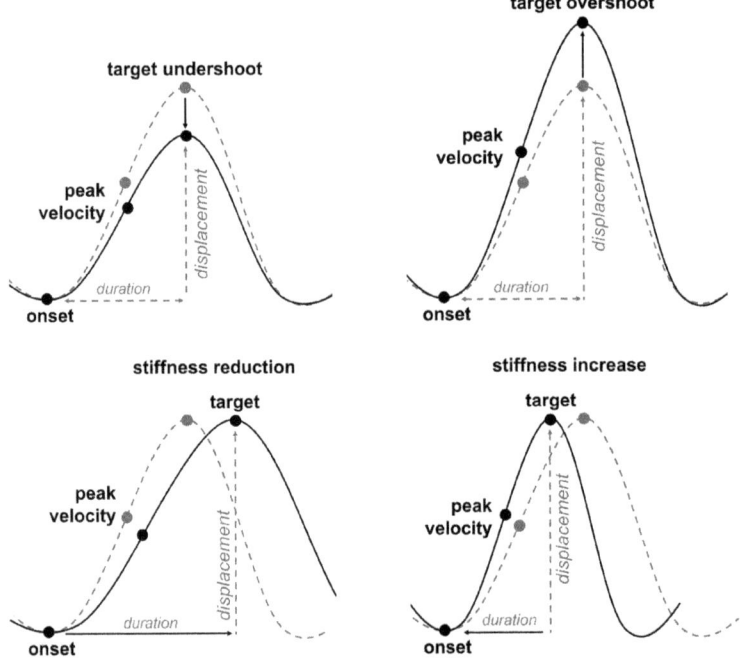

Figure 3.6. Articulatory modification possibilities. Top row: Target modification. Bottom row: Stiffness modification. Figure adapted from Mücke (2018).

Modification of Stiffness

A modification of stiffness changes the temporal orientation of a movement (Figure 3.6, bottom row). As stiffness is a parameter that refers to the relative speed of a movement, reducing or increasing it will change the oscillation frequency and therefore the time a movement needs to achieve its target (Ostry & Munhall, 1985). As a result, amplitude remains the same, but the total movement duration and speed change. A stiffness reduction leads to slower and longer movements, and an increased stiffness shortens and speeds up the movement (Munhall et al., 1985).

Modification of Target Height and Stiffness

Another modification option is the rescaling of time and space evoked by a proportional change of the target height and the stiffness. In this scenario, both amplitude and duration either increse or decrease simultaneously, while peak velocity remains unchanged.

Modifications do not change temporal and spatial characteristics alone, because changes in underlying articulatory movements can also be reflected in the acoustic output with regard to the quantity or quality of a sound. Longer and slower movements lead to longer acoustic segment durations, while smaller and faster movements shorten the segment duration. In addition, so-called hyper-articulation or hypo-articulation can change the sound (Lindblom, 1990). Smaller movements in terms of an articulatory undershoot can lead to a change in the sound quality, as the aimed target is not achieved. For example, if the plosive [t] is to be articulated but its target position consisting of a full closure is not reached, the listener may perceive the fricative [s] instead of the plosive [t]. In contrast, the articulation can also be particularly distinct and precise, resulting in larger movements and sometimes a target overshoot (Lindblom, 1990).

As shown above, the AP/TD model is capable of describing movement patterns when specific parameters are altered (Saltzman & Munhall, 1989; Saltzman, 1986). Speech parameters are modified, for example, in compensatory articulation. Some reasons for compensation in speech will be described below.

3.3.1 Compensation Strategies

Conversations can take place under normal communicative circumstances as well as under challenging conditions. Challenges can be caused due to, inter alia, environmental disturbances (noise), the listener (hearing loss) or physiological conditions of the speaker (aging or disease leading to deviant speech). To overcome these challenges, speakers need to change the way they speak, so that the listener nevertheless perceives the intended information. This indicates that speech is not only goal-directed with respect to articulatory target achievement, but also listener-oriented.

The process of speech production is aimed at an intelligible speech output that is understood by the listener. To achieve this auditory goal, speakers adapt their output along a continuum of hyper-articulation on the one side and hypo-articulation on the other side (Lindblom, 1990). According to Lindblom's H&H theory, a speaker wants to be understood as much as possible, but at the same time make the least possible effort. While, hypo-articulation is reflected in less distinct articulation, more overlap between movements and lower speech effort, hyper-articulation is reflected in more distinct articulation, less overlap between movements, and overall higher speech effort.

It has been shown that compensation strategies in most often cases lead to hyper-articulation. Speakers adapt to new requirements driven by internal or external factors to maintain their goal-directed speech production and thus accept having to invest more articulatory energy if needed. In general, using clear speech is a strategy for which acoustic-phonetic parameters are modulated to compensate for constraining factors (Mattys et al., 2012). To achieve clear speech, speakers reduce their speech rate and increase their pause frequency and intensity level compared to their normal speaking behavior, for the sake of intelligibility. As per H&H model, this is referred to as hyper-articulation (Lindblom, 1990). Especially in noisy environments, speakers speak louder in order to be understood (Folk & Schiel, 2011).

However, speakers may also adjust the position of their articulators and the coordination of speech movements (Gracco & Abbs, 1988). In a study by Brunner, Hoole, Perrier, and Fuchs (2006) speakers wore a prosthesis that changed the shape of the palate for a period of two weeks. The subjects adapted to the perturbed palate shape by lowering and retracting the tongue to produce intelligible speech output again. Other previous studies provide insights into the aging process with regard to physiological changes that affect the speech system. It has been observed for older speakers that movement durations of the tongue body increase with age (Thies et al., 2022; Mücke et al., 2021; Hermes et al., 2018). This prolongation is especially reflected in longer deceleration phases and more asymmetrical movement patterns. A slowdown of speech production can change the ratio of acceleration and deceleration phases (Ostry et al., 1987) and is further reflected in multiple velocity peaks that indicate submovements. A recent paper confirms that older adults also show slower limb movements and states further that they employ more submovements for goal-directed pointing movements, indicating less accurate movement patterns (Kornatz et al., 2021). Submovements are presumably attempts to achieve the articulatory goal, as it has been shown that the articulatory target was stable timed with respect to the acoustic syllable (Thies et al., 2022). Thus, the observed pattern can be interpreted as a compensatory strategy to counteract age effects on speech planning, allowing articulatory targets to be reached at the right time (Mücke et al., 2021; Hermes et al., 2018).

Depending on how long the challenging condition lasts, it may take some time for speakers to adapt to it (Löfqvist, 2010). With regard to this, Brunner et al. (2006) showed that different stages of adaptation arise, the longer speakers have to deal with the new demands. This applies to speakers who have to adapt to changing physical conditions as they get older or develop a disease: They have to learn to deal with possible deviations in order to produce targeted speech movements (Thies et al., 2022). However, compensation mechanisms involving underlying articulatory movements do not necessarily result in different speech output, as articulatory targets can be achieved in different ways (Perrier & Fuchs, 2015).

3.3.2 Prominence Marking

Modifications can also be task-specific (Löfqvist, 2010), for instance in the case of prosodic prominence marking. Prominence marking is a strategy to highlight specific parts within an utterance to make them stand out in comparison to others. Moreover, highlighting directs the listeners' attention to important information to ensure that the intended meaning of the utterance is conveyed. One specific function of prominence is to indicate the information structure of an utterance by means of focus marking

(Lambrecht, 1996). Within a communicative context, already given information is classified as less important and thus not highlighted on the acoustic surface (not prominent), while new or less accessible information is made prominent via accentuation (Gussenhoven, 2004).

The examples below (taken from Roessig, Winter, & Mücke, 2022, p. 2) clarify what is referred to by elements being in *focus* and *background* condition. Focused constituents are indicated by a subscripted F; information in background position by a subscripted B. The question-answer-scenario given in example (1) presents a so-called *broad focus* condition. In this focus condition, the whole answer is focused, since all information given in the response is assumed to be new to the listener and therefore highlighted. In contrast, in example (2) the girl name Mary is in *contrastive focus* condition, which means that the constituent is focused and serves as a correction of the name given in the question (Jane - Mary). The rest of the utterance contains given information and is shifted to the *background* position. As these examples show, the focus domain becomes smaller from broad focus to contrastive focus.

(1) *Broad focus*
Q: What's new? - A: [Nora wants to meet Mary.]$_F$

(2) *Contrastive focus*
Q: Does Nora wants to meet Jane? - A: [Nora wants to meet]$_B$ [Mary.]$_F$

(3) *'Mary' in out-of focus position*
Q: Who wants to meet Mary? - A: [Nora]$_F$ [wants to meet Mary.]$_B$

Three conditions are relevant for this work: background, broad focus, and contrastive focus. While, background is classified as non-prominent and out-of-focus, broad and contrastive focus are classified as prominent, in-focus conditions, with a higher degree of prominence found in the latter. Pitch accents are usually placed on target words in-focus condition to generate prominence. The degree of prosodic adjustments increases from non-prominent to prominent constituents, so that the perceived prominence increases along with it (Figure 3.7). The distinction between background and in-focus conditions, such as broad focus, is considered a comparison *across accentuation*. Differentiating between the in-focus types, such as broad focus and contrastive focus, is considered a comparison of degrees of contrast *within accentuation*. In general, prosodic adjustments and therefore the degree of prominence increase from background to broad focus and further to contrastive focus condition (Roessig & Mücke, 2019; Hermes et al., 2008; Baumann et al., 2007). However, a recent paper postulates that prosodic adjustments are more subtle within accentuation (Roessig et al., 2022).

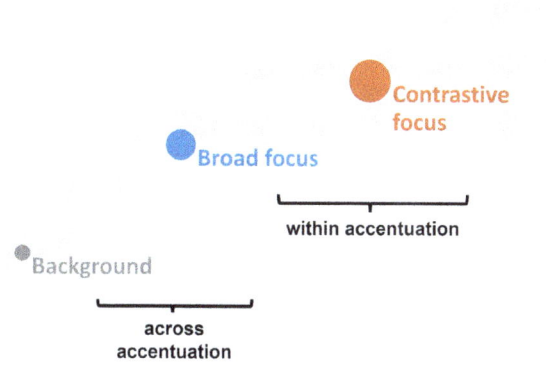

Figure 3.7. Increasing degrees of prosodic adjustments from background to broad focus and further to contrastive focus.

Speech production is adjusted for producing prominence in order to differentiate focus types along the continuum of non-prominent to prominent. Prosodic prominence is a complex process that requires sophisticated speech motor control, as all speech systems are involved. Prominence is realized by adjusting multiple phonetic cues, such as variation in fundamental frequency (speech melody, perceived pitch), intensity (perceived loudness), and articulatory features. In non-prominent positions, the physical control system tends to minimize the amount of articulatory effort for the different subsystems involved (Mattingly, 1981), a low-cost strategy, which is related to hypo-articulation (Lindblom, 1990). Hyper-articulation, in contrast, leads to an increase of articulatory effort to signal prominence.

In West Germanic languages, such as German, information structure assigns prosodic prominence. Thus, the underlying focus structure determines which word or which part of an utterance is focused. Especially stressed syllables can function as a domain for prosodic modifications. As mentioned above, prosodic adjustments involve all subsystems of speech to increase or decrease the perceived prominence. Figure 3.8 presents increasing intensity values and syllable durations as well as stronger modulation of fundamental frequency (F0) from left to right, from unaccented to accented conditions. These adjustments are gradient and categorical in nature (Baumann et al., 2006) and will be described below.

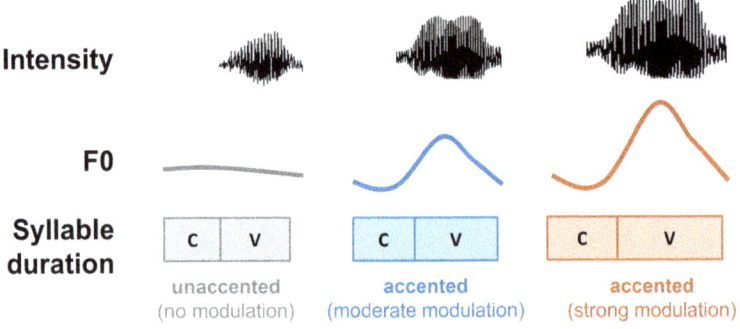

Figure 3.8. Expected changes for prominence marking on the acoustic level.

In the respiratory system, prominence is associated with an increase in subglottal pressure, which leads to an increase in perceived loudness. The acoustic correlate of loudness is the intensity level, which is often measured in decibel (dB). Higher intensity values are found in accented, prominent syllables. However, the role of intensity as a primary marker of prominence is under debate, as some studies report it as contributing to prominence (Harrington et al., 2000; Lowit et al., 2018; Fowler, 1995), whereas another sees it contributing only to a small extent (Kochanski et al., 2005). Modifications of intensity seem to be especially relevant across accentuation, but only slightly within accentuation (Roessig et al., 2022).

Modifications within the phonatory system are related to pitch changes that occur on prominent syllables in particular (Ladd, 2008; Gussenhoven, 2004; van Heuven & Sluijter, 1996). Changes in pitch result in tones that are perceived by the listener as pitch accents. According to the autosegmental-metrical model of intonation, these tones can be classified into different pitch accent types. Depending on the characteristics of each pitch accent, the degree of perceived prominence varies, as several pitch accents differ in their pitch height, their movement direction and their alignment within the tone-bearing syllable.

With regard to pitch height, higher pitch peaks are perceived as more prominent (Roessig, 2021; Baumann & Röhr, 2015; Gussenhoven, 2004) and seem to be important to differentiate across accentuation (Roessig et al., 2022). Moreover, rising pitch contours are overall more prominent than falling pitch contours (Röhr et al., 2020; Baumann & Winter, 2018; Baumann & Röhr, 2015; Braun & Ladd, 2003). In addition, steeper movements towards the pitch peak are perceived as more prominent as well (Baumann & Röhr, 2015). Another parameter is the alignment of the pitch target to the tone-bearing syllable: Later peak alignment is perceived as more prominent (Roessig, 2021; Baumann & Grice, 2006; Kohler, 1991) and used to distinguish prominence within accentuation (Roessig et al., 2022). Pitch changes are shown to be the strongest correlate of prominence and thus reliable for the listener to perceive different degrees of prominence (Roessig et al., 2022; Baumann & Winter, 2018; Ladd, 2008).

Prominence involves speakers modulating articulatory features as well. Especially the vocalic part of a syllable is subject to prosodic modifications, while the role of consonants is still being contested (Mücke, 2018; Cho, 2006; Cho & McQueen, 2005; Fougeron & Keating, 1997). Articulation becomes more clear and distinct (van Heuven & Sluijter, 1996), with two forms of modification strategies being applied: *sonority expansion* and *hyper-articulation*. Both strategies often go hand in hand with each other. However, a recent study suggests, that the strategy of hyper-articulation is favored by listeners (Steffman, 2021).

Sonority expansion refers to more acoustic energy radiating from the mouth, increasing the perceived prominence degree (De Jong et al., 1993; Beckman et al., 1992). Sonority is enhanced by increasing durational properties, allowing longer acoustic segments or syllables to be determined under prominence, which are usually measured in milliseconds (Roessig et al., 2022; Mücke & Grice, 2016; Kügler, 2008; Baumann et al., 2007, 2006; Braun & Ladd, 2003; Beckman et al., 1992). Another way to enhance sonority is to increase the degree of opening of the oral cavity (Harrington et al., 2000; Cho, 2006, 2005). However, it can be difficult to distinguish this strategy from hyper-articulation (De Jong, 1995; Lindblom, 1990), as the latter involves more distinct vocal tract configurations, which lead to an enlargement of the overall vowel space (Kent & Kim, 2003) or more opening.

Hyper-articulation increases paradigmatic contrasts between constituents. To enhance perceptual contrasts, the articulatory effort is increased, leading to a more distinct production of segments, syllables, or words (Nelson & Wedel, 2017; Mücke & Grice, 2014; Scarborough, 2013; Harrington et al., 2000; Baese-Berk & Goldrick, 2009; Cho, 2005; De Jong, 1995). More extreme tongue positions that are articulated when producing vowels under prominence are reflected in changes in vowel formant frequencies (Baumann et al., 2007). Vocalic movements are adjusted not only in the vertical dimension (open-closed), but also in the horizontal domain (front-back) to achieve a vocalic target on the periphery. For example, the tongue body is more fronted when producing a prominent /i/, or more retracted when producing a prominent /o/. Configurations in this front-back dimension change the vowel formant F2: Frequencies of F2 are supposed to be higher for prominent /i/ and lower for prominent /o/. With regard to the open-closed dimension, a prominent /a/ is articulated with a much more lowered tongue and a greater jaw opening, increasing vowel formant F1. Thus, more peripheral vowel formant frequencies can be measured, indicating an extension of the overall articulation space under prominence (Kent & Kim, 2003).

Articulatory changes do not only occur on the acoustic level, but also on underlying articulatory movements of the lips and the tongue. As Figure 3.9 illustrates, movements are longer and larger under prominence (Thies et al., 2022; Katsika, 2018; Mücke & Grice, 2014; Hermes et al., 2008; Cho, 2006; Harrington et al., 2000; De Jong, 1995; Beckman et al., 1992). Thus, articulatory movements are rescaled in time and space (cf. Section 3.3). It has been shown in previous studies that the degree of lip opening during vowel production is modulated for different focus conditions in German and English (Krivokapić et al., 2017; Mücke & Grice, 2014; Hermes et al., 2008). Lip aperture increases across accentuation and within accentuation. The same pattern was observed for tongue body movements in healthy German speakers, as tongue positions and movement velocities were systematically adjusted across accentuation and within accentuation (Pagel et al., 2020; Roessig & Mücke, 2019).

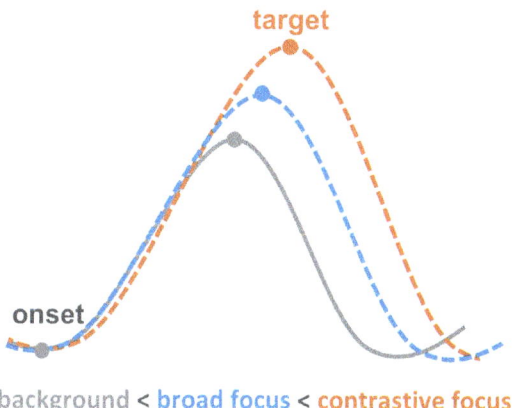

Figure 3.9. Expected changes for prominence marking on the articulatory level.

However it seems that articulatory changes are especially relevant to differentiate modulations across accentuation, as changes within accentuation are more subtle (Roessig et al., 2022). This is probably due to the fact that articulation is already particular distinct and extreme, leaving hardly any room to move the articulators further to the periphery, in order to be differentiated within accentuation (Roessig et al., 2022).

All movement patterns reported above were observed in healthy speakers. But as already mentioned, changes in the physiological conditions of a speaker due to aging or disease can change speech production on different levels, e.g. respiration, articulation, and phonation. As (speech) motor control decreases with age or specific diseases (Thies et al., 2022; Kornatz et al., 2021; Mücke et al., 2021; Duffy, 2019; Hermes et al., 2018), the question arises what happens to speech if motor control is affected. The next chapter describes speech pattern that can be observed in speakers with Parkinson's disease, a patient cohort that suffer from reduced motor functions.

4 Speech in Parkinson's Disease

4.1 Hypokinetic Dysarthria

A speech disorder is characterized by deviations in the speech motor process from planning to execution (cf. Chapter 3.1). One type of speech disorder is the so-called dysarthria, which accounts for 50 % of all speech disorders (cf. Duffy, 2019, p. 6). Dysarthria is a neurological disorder and is generally caused by damage to the nervous system. It is often accompanied by a movement disorder affecting the speed, range, and accuracy of speech movements. Different types of dysarthria are distinguished: flaccid, spastic, ataxic, hyperkinetic, and hypokinetic (Duffy, 2019). Mixed types may also occur.

Hypokinetic dysarthria is the type of dysarthria that is induced by PD. It is related to the neural motor system and is associated with affected basal ganglia circuits that impact speech motor control (cf. Section 2.1.2). The deficits in speech motor control inhibit the preparation and maintenance of motor programs but also the ability to switch between them (Spencer & Rogers, 2005). This leads to a hypo-functionality of the speech system in terms of reduced muscular forces and movements, and a reduced control over fine motor skills. Up to 90 % of patients with PD develop this kind of dysarthria in the course of the disease (Duffy, 2019; Müller et al., 2001). The manifestation of dysarthric symptoms is highly individual but consistently stable within a patient (Yorkston et al., 1988). A strong manifestation often occurs at later stages of the disease. However, deviant underlying speech mechanisms cause less intelligible and less natural speech compared to non-deviant speech, and negatively affect the patients' ability to communicate.

4.1.1 Intelligibility and Naturalness

Early approaches to characterizing dysarthrias are based on auditory-perceptual classifications (Darley et al., 1969). The work of Darley et al. (1969) was fundamental for today's knowledge of dysarthrias as well as their diverse representations and distinct types with salient features.

Especially in clinical contexts, the diagnosis of speech disorders is still based on perceptual ratings, since instrumental methods or tools are rare and time-consuming. Such ratings are therefore rather subjective and rater-specific. One promising objective and cost-effective alternative could be the use of automatic speech signal analysis in the future (Baghai-Ravary & Beet, 2012), such as *the dysarthria analyzer* (Hlavnicka, 2018) or the *MonPaGe screening protocol* (Laganaro et al., 2021). In both approaches, acoustic speech samples are recorded by following a short protocol of standard speech production tasks. The analysis of distinctive acoustic speech features might be practicable in the clinical routine.

However, many studies investigating speech in PD report ratings of *intelligibility* and/or *naturalness* (Klopfenstein, 2016; Stipancic et al., 2016; Anand & Stepp, 2015; Tjaden et al., 2014; Kempler & van Lancker, 2002). In this context, intelligibility often refers to the amount of words understood by the listener, and rarely to the listeners' effort. Either clinicians or naive listeners rate the intelligibility of patients' speech output (Duffy, 2019). Naturalness, in contrast, describes whether the speech conforms to the listener's expectations of natural, unimpaired speech (Yorkston et al., 1999). It is reflected in the speakers' prosody in terms of speech rate, voice quality, and loudness (Klopfenstein et al., 2020).

Ratings are often made by means of a Likert scale, a visual analog scale, an orthographic transcription or by using categorical classifications (Stipancic et al., 2021; Hirsch et al., 2022; Lehner et al., 2021; Klopfenstein, 2016; Stipancic et al., 2016; Klopfenstein, 2015; Landa et al., 2014; Cote-Reschny & Hodge, 2010; Whitehill & Wong, 2006; Onslow et al., 1992). Each approach is far away from having a consistent methodology (Stipancic et al., 2021; Klopfenstein et al., 2020), but if a speech disorder is present, there seems to be high inter-rater consistency regarding ratings concerning the severity of the dysarthria (Stipancic et al., 2021). Therefore, perceptual ratings can be seen as reliable indicator for the presence of hypokinetic dysarthria, although they rely on subjective judgments, which may vary across raters, and prevent varying levels of naturalness or intelligibility from being assessed.

Furthermore, these ratings reflect whether and to what extent the dysarthria has an impact on the patients' daily life. This knowledge is essential, as patients aim to be understood by other people in social communicative contexts. Participation in everyday life is aggravated by incomprehensible speech and is made even more difficult if patients are stigmatized based on their way of speaking (Hertrich et al., 2021). For example, patients who speak slowly and slurred all the time might be perceived as intoxicated. Especially spontaneous speech, which represents most of daily communication is rated as less intelligible (Weir-Mayta et al., 2017; Kempler & van Lancker, 2002) and also least natural (Klopfenstein, 2016) in speakers with dysarthria compared to reading or repetition.

Tackling the impact of dysarthria on everyday life should be a key element of treatment management in patients with dysarthria (WHO, 2001). Especially reduced intelligibility seems to be accompanied by an increased severity of dysarthria (Tjaden et al., 2014). Therefore, the common goal of speech therapy is to increase speech intelligibility. However, increased intelligibility can lead to decreased naturalness and vice versa. So the challenge is to balance these two aims and adjust the therapy to train the best possible way of speaking.

The following speech dimensions are mainly affected by hypokinetic dysarthria: pitch modulation, loudness variation, voice quality, imprecise articulation, speaking rate, and pausing behavior (Duffy, 2019; Darley et al., 1975). Changes in one or more of these speech dimensions can lead to less intelligible and rather unnatural speech in speakers with PD. The deviations that may occur in these perceptual speech characteristics are discussed in more detail in the following subchapters.

4.1.2 Respiratory-Phonatory Control

Respiration

As a consequence of a hypokinesia of the respiratory musculature, patients with PD experience a reduction in breath support, lower lung pressure and therefore shorter expiratory cycles (Hertrich et al., 2021). This in turn leads to shorter phrase length and a higher amount of inappropriately placed pauses (Skodda, 2015; Ziegler & Vogel, 2010). Reduced breath support diminishes the energy that radiates from the mouth (cf. Chapter 3.1) and lowers measurable intensity values. The consequence is reduced loudness (Delvaux et al., 2018) and quiet speech (Walsh & Smith, 2012), which is a typical symptom of speech production in PD (Duffy, 2019). To investigate the respiratory system and to capture the reduced breath support, intensity values are calculated in various tasks as they are correlated with perceived loudness.

Respiratory capacity is typically measured by looking at the maximum phonation of vowels, such as /a/ and /i/ in order to examine the prolonged activation of respiratory and laryngeal muscles (Rosen et al., 2005). Speech of individuals with PD is characterized by shorter maximum phonation times, accompanied by lower intensity values indicating quieter speech production (de Keyser et al., 2016). Moreover, it has been shown that speakers with PD are less able to maintain consistent intensity levels in different tasks, such as reading, uttering a monologue (Rusz et al., 2011) or in fast syllable repetition tasks (Rosen et al., 2005). This decay over time is described as hypophonia.

To increase overall speech loudness, patients are trained to increase vocal effort. It has been shown that speech treatments, such as the Lee Silverman Voice Treatment (LSVT LOUD; Fox, Ebersbach, Ramig, & Sapir, 2012), which is precisely aimed at improving respiratory support and strengthening laryngeal muscles in speakers with PD, yield positive results that can be maintained for about two years (Ramig et al., 2001).

Phonation

The phonatory function refers to the glottal activity of the vocal folds. Especially voicing is an active control process of vocal fold abduction. In speakers with PD, the rigor in laryngeal muscles impacts this phonatory control (Duffy, 2019). Impaired phonatory control leads to changes in voice quality on the one hand, and a reduced ability to modulate pitch on the other hand.

The voice quality of speakers with PD is described as harsh and breathy (Hertrich et al., 2021; Duffy, 2019), sometimes accompanied by a vocal tremor. This is due to incomplete closures of the vocal folds and incorrect vocal fold oscillations (Rusz et al., 2011), which is summarized under the term hypophonia. Reduced phonatory control can be observed in the production of stop consonants, as intended voiceless stops become (partly) voiced (Rusz et al., 2011). Conversely, a devoicing of intended voiced stop consonants is also reported (Antolík & Fougeron, 2013). Both phenomena indicate a poor coordination between glottal and oral control (Kent et al., 1999).

Vocal fold control also affects pitch in terms of pitch height and pitch modulation. Previous research reports on decreased variation of fundamental frequency in speakers with impaired vocal fold control (Hsu et al., 2017; de Keyser et al., 2016; Rusz et al., 2011; Skodda, Grönheit, & Schlegel, 2011). Furthermore, Skodda and colleagues report a reduction in variability of the fundamental frequency throughout a reading task, indicating a decay over time. Thus, the same phenomenon reported for intensity is reported for fundamental frequency. The reduction in variability tends to deteriorate with disease duration (Skodda, Grönheit, & Schlegel, 2011).

To sum up, speakers with PD have reduced control over the phonatory-respiratory system. This is clearly observable in terms of quieter speech and reduced modulation of pitch and loudness, which can lead to monopitch and monoloudness in advanced hypokinetic dysarthria. Monotonous speech indicates an impaired ability to convey (prosodic) stress patterns. This will be described in section 4.1.5.

4.1.3 Articulation

Articulatory deficits concern consonantal and vocalic sounds (Duffy, 2019). As previous studies have shown, reduced intelligibility in speakers with PD arises from impaired articulatory skills (Thies et al., 2020; Duffy, 2019; Delvaux et al., 2018; Antolík & Fougeron, 2013; Skodda, Visser, & Schlegel, 2011; Kim et al., 2011; McRae et al., 2002).

Specifically, articulatory deficits in speakers with PD are thought to result in less accurate articulation caused by the generally reduced articulatory working space, which is associated with smaller (and slower) movements of the tongue, lips, and jaw (Kearney et al., 2017; Duffy, 2019). Reduced articulatory movement amplitudes seem to be responsible for reducing intelligibility in speakers with PD (Kearney et al., 2017; Kim et al., 2011; Forrest et al., 1989). Consequently, larger speech movement amplitudes have been shown to result in intelligibility gains in these speakers (Kearney et al., 2017). Therefore, the common goal of therapeutic interventions is to increase the amplitude of speech movements.

Whether the movement speed has an influence on speech intelligibility is currently unclear.

Consonants

Already in 1981, Logemann and Fisher (1981) found the articulation of consonants in speakers with PD to be imprecise. The imprecision is due to a failure to achieve the articulatory target of a full closure in the production of stop consonants (Hertrich et al., 2021; Duffy, 2019; Ackermann & Ziegler, 1991). Incomplete closures result further in spirantization and a more noisy acoustic speech signal because friction is produced during the intended full closure.

Previous acoustic studies recorded speakers performing either fast syllable repetition or sentence production tasks to capture deviant productions of stop consonants. A study by Karlsson and Hartelius (2019) asserts that articulatory imprecision is best captured in tasks using syllable repetitions of /ka-ka-ka/, as the velar place of articulation is the first to be affected by hypokinetic dysarthria. Another study postulates that misarticulations of consonantal sounds seem to correlate with axial symptoms (Rusz, Tykalová, Novotnỳ, et al., 2021). The imprecisions may be counterbalanced with a clear or louder speaking style (Tjaden & Martel-Sauvageau, 2017), since corresponding treatment approaches are associated with increased movement amplitudes (Mefferd, 2017; Darling & Huber, 2011; Dromey, 2000).

Vowels

Regarding vowel articulation, literature reports an overall reduced vowel space and a centralization of formant frequencies (McRae et al., 2002; Weismer et al., 2001). Vowel formant frequencies are mostly used as a measure of articulatory configurations of the tongue. The vowel formant F1 represents the vertical tongue position (tongue height, raised vs. lowered), while the vowel formant F2 represents the horizontal tongue position (tongue advancement, front vs. back; Kent et al., 1999). Reduced F2 slopes are mentioned in previous research indicating difficulties with tongue configurations along the horizontal axis (Weismer et al., 2012); often measured when diphthongs were produced (Lansford & Liss, 2014; Walsh & Smith,

Hypokinetic Dysarthria 69

2012; Kim et al., 2011, 2009). In line with this, a more centralized production of the vowels /u/ and /o/, revealed by higher values of the vowel formant F2, was observed in speakers with PD (Thies et al., 2020; Rusz, Cmejla, Tykalová, et al., 2013).

Smaller acoustic vowel spaces are illustrated in most studies (Thies et al., 2022; Hsu et al., 2017; Whitfield & Goberman, 2014; Rusz, Cmejla, Tykalová, et al., 2013; Rusz et al., 2011; Sapir et al., 2010, 2003; McRae et al., 2002; Weismer et al., 2001); either in the form of plotted vowel space areas or calculated ratios by using vowel formants F1 and F2. One way of measuring the latter is to calculate the Euclidean distances in a quadrilateral space between vowel formants F1 and F2 of /i/, /æ/, /a/, and /u/ (Kent & Kim, 2003), or within a triangular vowel space space between the vowels /a/, /i/, and /u/. While most of the results point in the same direction, a study by Delvaux et al. (2018) found no difference in vowel space between healthy controls and patients with PD using the calculation of Euclidean distance.

Another option is the calculation of the so-called *Vowel Articulation Index*. It is preferred over the previous measurement due to its sensitivity to highly variable data, making it more suitable for detecting changes in vowel articulation in dysarthric speech (Skodda et al., 2012; Skodda, Visser, & Schlegel, 2011; Sapir et al., 2010; Roy et al., 2009). Smaller values represent a decreased vowel space which is reported in a number of studies for speakers with PD (Thies et al., 2022, 2020; Skodda et al., 2012; Skodda, Visser, & Schlegel, 2011).

The reduction of acoustic vowel contrast seems to relate to tongue-specific articulatory impairment in speakers with PD (Mefferd & Dietrich, 2019). Furthermore, the overall motor status may impact speech, as a higher degree of motor impairment correlates with a reduction and centralization of the vowel space (Thies et al., 2021, 2020). While Skodda et al. (2012) did not find a relationship between overall impairment and vowel space, they mention a relation with gait impairment; an axial symptom.

Acoustic vowel contrast can be increased by a clear speaking style, which is associated with an extension of the articulation space (Tjaden et al., 2013). In addition, acoustic studies reveal that a slower speech or articulation rate is associated with a larger acoustic space (McRae et al., 2002) and more distinct articulation (Fletcher et al., 2015), resulting in an increase of contrasts in the acoustic and perceptual space (hyper-articulation; cf. Chapter 3.3).

What can be measured on the acoustic level is based on underlying articulatory movements within the vocal tract. For vowel production in PD it was shown that the articulatory-to-acoustic relation is strong, indicating that changes of tongue movements, for instance in terms of movement range, can be related to acoustic vowel contrast (distance between two vowels in the articulatory space) (Mefferd, 2015). Therefore, studies investigating speech kinematics will be presented in the following subchapter.

4.1.4 Underlying Kinematics

Duffy (2019) describes that speech movements in PD are reduced in the temporal and spatial dimension. They are slower, less flexible, less extended (reduced range or amplitude), and exhibit scaling problems with regard to both dimensions amplitude and duration (Duffy, 2019). While the slowness of the articulators is attributed to PD-related bradykinesia, the reduced range and speed is concomitant to hypokinesia. A common term used in the context of describing speech in PD is *articulatory undershoot*, which refers to the fact that an articulatory movement fails to reach its target (Hertrich et al., 2021; Darley et al., 1975). The articulatory undershooting thereby depends on the speaking rate (Hertrich & Ackermann, 2017; McRae et al., 2002).

So far, only a few studies examined the underlying speech movements in the articulatory domain that are responsible for what can be measured as speech properties on the acoustic level (Kearney et al., 2017; Bandini et al., 2016; Walsh & Smith, 2012). Temporal and spatial modifications of articulatory movements underlie changes in syllable or word production in speech. While temporal modifications relate to changes in movement duration (shorter or longer movements), spatial modifications refer to changes in the amplitude of a movement (smaller or larger displacements; cf. Chapter 3.3). Depending on how spatial and temporal parameters are modified, the speed of the movement changes as well (faster or slower movements). Previous kinematic studies directly tracked movements of the jaw, lips, tongue tip, and tongue body during speech by using methods such as electromagnetic articulography or X-ray microbeams. The results will be reported below for each articulator separately.

Lip and Jaw Movement

Most of the studies agree that lip and jaw movements are overall reduced in speakers with PD. Two studies investigated orofacial movements during natural sentence production in parkinsonian speech (Kearney et al., 2017; Walsh & Smith, 2012). They reported reduced lip movements in the spatial domain along with reduced velocities for patients compared to healthy controls. Also, shorter lip amplitude without durational change was found in repetitions of the syllable /va/ by Connor, Abbs, Cole, and Gracco (1989). A recent study underlines the reduction in lip amplitude and reduced movement speed in speakers with PD compared to healthy controls, also highlighting that movement durations, stiffness, and time-to-peak are comparable across speaker groups (Kim et al., 2021).

Another study describes lip movements during consonant production to be smaller in amplitude as well as shorter in duration in two native Italian speakers with PD compared to two healthy control speakers (Fivela et al., 2014). A study by Forrest and Weismer (1995) differentiates opening and closing lip movements, demonstrating that durational properties depend on movement direction, as movement durations were the same for parkinsonian and healthy speakers in opening gestures, but shorter in closing movements in speakers with PD. However, they also report reduced displacements and peak velocities (Forrest & Weismer, 1995). A small study explores smaller but longer closing movements of the lower lip in productions of bilabial stops in speakers with PD (Thompson, 2018). Two other studies observe slower but not smaller lip movements in sentence production (Yunusova et al., 2008) and fast syllable repetition tasks of /pa-pa-pa/ (Bandini et al., 2016). Slower movements need more time to reach the same target in terms of amplitude, resulting in longer movement durations.

In parallel to the findings for lip movements, reduced amplitude and velocity was also reported for jaw movements in speakers with PD compared to control speakers (Kearney et al., 2017; Walsh & Smith, 2012; Robertson et al., 2011; Connor et al., 1989), albeit with comparable, constant movement durations.

Tongue Movement

Tongue movements can be involved in consonantal or vocalic sounds. One study investigated tongue movements during the production of alveolar and velar consonants (Wong et al., 2011). It compared dysarthric patients with PD, non-dysarthric patients with PD, and healthy controls. When comparing PD patients with and without dysarthria, temporal differences in terms of faster and shorter movements were found for the consonants in the dysarthria group. However, when comparing patients with dysarthria to healthy controls, patients performed with larger, longer, and faster tongue movements. In contrast, patients without dysarthria produced smaller, slower, and longer tongue movements compared to healthy controls. This study questions the assumption of reduced speech movements in dysarthric speakers with PD in terms of consonantal weakening.

So far, not much is known about tongue kinematics in parkinsonian speech during vowel production. This is surprising, since the acoustic vowel space was reported to be reduced in several previous studies. Focusing on the spatial domain, tongue closing movements during vowel productions were larger in two patients compared to healthy controls (Fivela et al., 2014). These results also question the assumption of reduced movement amplitudes for speech movements in PD. But it should be considered that patient data showed a very heterogeneous pattern on the articulatory level ranging from hyper- to hypo-articulation within and across speakers, as reported by the authors. A study by Mefferd (2015) observed smaller tongue displacements in productions of the diphthong /ai/ in the word "kite".

In the temporal domain, similar durations but slower speeds of tongue body movements were reported during vowel production (Yunusova et al., 2008). An exploratory study with a small sample size, observed longer tongue body movement durations and longer deceleration phases in speakers with PD (Thies et al., 2022), leading to asymmetrical velocity profiles of speech movements. A prolongation of the deceleration phase has been interpreted as an indicator for dysarthric speech (Ziegler, 2002; Kent et al., 2000; Ackermann et al., 1995; Forrest & Weismer, 1995), suggesting a reorganization of the movement strategies in speakers with dysarthria. However, a recent paper states that submovements (based on multiple velocity peaks) also occur in elderly adults in goal-directed pointing movements, indicating less accurate movement patterns and changing velocity profiles (Kornatz et al., 2021). The same tendency for longer deceleration phases was reported for speech of older speakers and speakers with PD by Thies et al. (2022). Therefore, deviations in gross motor performance can also be found in speech motor performance.

However, prolongation in deceleration phases can also be interpreted as a compensation strategy to achieve the articulatory target at the right time, as shown in a study by Thies et al. (2022). In terms of timing relations, the vocalic target was achieved at a stable point in time, whereas the movement initiation was rather variable across all speaker groups (older, younger, PD) and overall earlier in speakers with PD. Findings confirming the stable coordination of vocalic targets were presented by Yunusova et al. (2008), who report similar timing measures between speakers with PD and healthy controls as well as preserved timing relations due to proportional changes in the interarticulator timing, such as between the lip and the tongue dorsum (Weismer et al., 2003).

Overall, larger effects of dysarthria on movements can be expected in the production of low vowels, as they require larger, longer, and faster movements (Yunusova et al., 2008). To sum up, most studies report underlying articulatory movements to be smaller in amplitude and slower in velocity in speakers with PD, indicating a down scaling in these domains. Decreased intelligibility is associated especially, with the reduction in movement amplitudes (Kearney et al., 2017).

4.1.5 Prosodic Characteristics

As described above in section 3.3.2, acoustic correlates of prosody are the relative segment duration and modulation of intensity and fundamental frequency. Taking all the above-mentioned domains of speech deviations in PD together, speakers with PD can be assumed to have difficulties modulating prosodic structures and problems conveying meanings appropriately.

Although the terms dysprosody, monopitch, and monoloudness are often reported in the context of PD, studies on prominence marking are rare.

It has been shown that modulation of prosodic phonetic features can be impaired in patients with PD (Duffy, 2019) or at least vary between speakers with PD and healthy controls (Tykalová et al., 2014; Azevedo et al., 2013; Cheang & Pell, 2007). With regard to focus marking (cf. Section 3.3.2), these deficits become visible when speakers with PD are asked to produce different degrees of prominence. Fivela, Sallustio, Pede, and Patrocinio (2021) argued that contrastive stress has a higher functional load and it might be more challenging for speakers with PD to differentiate, for example, broad focus from contrastive focus. In line with this expectation, contrastive stress was not successfully communicated by speakers with PD, as it was not identifiable by listeners in a study by Pell, Cheang, and Leonard (2006).

However, in prosodically important positions, patients may be able to temporarily compensate for the distortion and produce the prosodic marking preserving the linguistic function (Antolík & Fougeron, 2013; Ackermann & Ziegler, 1991). A study shows that the prosodic function was preserved in 20 male Czech speakers with PD reading a text passage aloud (Tykalová et al., 2014). Unaccented and accented conditions could still be differentiated by parameters such as duration, intensity, and fundamental frequency (F0). However, speakers with PD modulated F0, intensity, and durational properties in prominent positions not to the same extent as the healthy control participants. These findings are supported by a recent study concluding that speakers with PD adjust F0, intensity, and vowel space in prominent positions, but the modifications are less effective or less distinct compared to control speakers (Thies et al., 2020).

In the following, disparities are described that shine a different light on the effectiveness of prominence marking. With regard to pitch modulation, speakers with PD produced fewer expected pitch contours in nuclear position in intonational phrases in comparison to healthy controls (Frota et al., 2021). They deviated in terms of more simplified pitch modulations (shallow rise vs. steep rise) or different directions of pitch movements (falling vs. rising). Reflecting this observation, earlier peaks and smaller amplitudes of pitch movements were observed in three female speakers of German with PD producing contrastive sentences and questions (Penner et al., 2001).

However, preserved patterns with regard to pitch have been reported as well, but with a tendency toward decreased contrasts in duration (Hertrich & Ackermann, 1993).

A sentence production experiment was conducted by Gaviria (2015), focusing on the three standard phonetic parameters and investigating vowel production with varying target word position. Results from 10 English speakers with PD demonstrated that they were able to use intensity and durational differences to signal prominence. While duration and intensity were used to the same degree for prominence marking comparing speakers with PD and control participants, speakers with PD differed from the control group as they did not adjust their vowel space and pitch contour. However, Thies et al. (2020) report that speakers with PD performed with a reduced vowel space in terms of hypo-articulated vowels, but hyper-articulated prosodic parameters, such as intensity and tonal range. Concerning loudness, Cheang and Pell (2007) found lower intensity values on prominent syllables in the production of 21 male and female native English speakers with PD when producing mini-dialogues.

On the articulatory level, prominence marking seems to be intact as speakers with PD produce longer, larger, and faster movements. But it is important to note that little research has been done so far.

A recent study by Kim et al. (2021) reports that prosodic marking is preserved on the articulatory level due to the fact that, besides overall reduced lip movements, speakers with PD produce longer movements, larger displacements, higher peak velocities, and lower stiffness in stressed conditions (Kim et al., 2021). Moreover, acceleration phases (time-to-peak) are prolonged in stressed conditions. By investigating not only lip but also jaw movements in stressed and unstressed syllables, Forrest and Weismer (1995) report reduced movement amplitudes and peak velocities for speakers with PD in both stressed and unstressed syllables. However, the relation between amplitude and velocity did not differ for the two groups for any movement. The same picture arises when determining strategies of word stress (e.g. meTROpoils, MAnicure), as speakers with PD show reduced amplitudes and velocities as well as shorter durations relative to healthy controls in both stress conditions (Forrest et al., 1989).

A small study focusing on tongue body movements during vowel production reports longer tongue movements in prominent positions

(Thies et al., 2022). While the control speakers marked prominence across and within accentuation, speakers with PD only differentiated between unaccented and accented productions without further differentiating for example broad focus from contrastive focus. A similar result was described by Thies et al. (2021), reporting that tongue body movements are adjusted in the temporal and spatial domain by speakers with PD, but only across accentuation.

All studies discussed above suggest that speakers with PD may experience problems at all levels of prominence marking. However, there seems to be great variation in both the affected phonetic parameter and the severity of the respective impairment. With regard to the reduced modulation of those parameters, Kent et al. (1999) remark that it is important to take variation into account, and claim that within-speaker-variation might be lower if the speech impairment is more severe.

4.1.6 Speech Rate and Fluency

The last parameter to be addressed is the speech rate. Rate refers to a measure that indicates a defined change or occurrence over time; for example, words per minute or syllables per second. To begin with, the difference between articulation rate and speaking rate will be clarified, as these two terms are sometimes used interchangeably. In contrast to the articulation rate, the speaking rate also takes pauses into account (Tsao et al., 2006). The articulation rate can also be measured in terms of syllable or pause duration (Liss et al., 2009).

Speakers with PD often speak at a normal speech rate (Hertrich et al., 2021). However, fluctuations in the rate pattern can be observed, as the speaking rate momentarily decreases or increases compared to healthy controls. Sometimes speech units partly include short rushes of speech that give the impression of an increased speaking rate (Duffy, 2019).

An overall slowing-down of speech rate is related to bradykinesia in PD and is usually measured in terms of syllables per second in fast syllable repetition or sentence production tasks. Prolonged syllables are described as an indicator of dysarthria (Ackermann et al., 1995). Patients with PD perform with slower rates when rapidly repeating syllable cycles, such as /pa-ta-ka/ (Rusz et al., 2011). Lower speech rates were also found when calculating the Inter-Syllabic Interval (Delvaux et al., 2018) and in reading tasks (Hsu et al., 2017). In contrast, studies report neither differences in terms of articulation rate (Lowit et al., 2006) nor regarding speech rate and syllable duration (Walsh & Smith, 2012; Ackermann & Ziegler, 1991) when comparing speakers with PD and healthy controls. Another study observed no differences in the overall speech rate, comparing healthy controls and patients with PD reading a standardized text. But the authors observed more syllables per second in patients with PD, and at the same time less and longer pauses leading to the impression of a hastened articulation (Skodda & Schlegel, 2008).

Dysfluencies may also occur in the speech of patients with PD, indicated by inappropriate pauses, increased pause times, and repetitions of syllables or words (Im et al., 2019; Goberman et al., 2005; Goberman & Blomgren, 2003).

4.2 Development of Speech Deficits

Hypokinetic dysarthria in PD appears to start with phonatory deficits and evolves further towards articulatory and fluency deficits (Hertrich & Ackermann, 2017; Ho et al., 1998). This progressive evolution from the larynx to posterior and later anterior lingual involvement, and eventually further to labial involvement was investigated in a study by Logemann, Fisher, Boshes, and Blonsky (1978), assessing the speech impairment of 200 patients:

- **Group 1:** Laryngeal dysfunction.
- **Group 2:** Laryngeal dysfunction and tongue back involvement.
- **Group 3:** Laryngeal, tongue back, and tongue blade dysfunction.
- **Group 4:** Laryngeal, tongue back, tongue blade dysfunction, and labial misarticulations.
- **Group 5:** Laryngeal dysfunction and misarticulations of the tongue back, tongue blade, lips, and tongue tip.

In line with this, Rusz, Cmejla, Tykalová, et al. (2013) assume that problems with tongue articulation develop from the tongue root to the tongue tip. This might be the reason why syllable repetitions in the velar region are a valid indicator of early speech deviations (Karlsson & Hartelius, 2019). Another study with a comparable sample size to the study of

Logemann et al. (1978) determined that there are speech clusters in PD that depend on a scaled severity of speech impairments (Ho et al., 1998) and cannot be captured by only rating their absence or presence in a binary fashion, as it has been done before by Logemann et al. (1978). However, this study supports the idea that reduced phonatory control is an early sign of hypokinetic dysarthria in PD and that articulatory impairments follow and gradually increase as speech deteriorates (Ho et al., 1998). It is therefore worthwhile to look for altered phonation in patients particularly early.

Table 4.1. Speech subtypes and their characteristics according to Rusz, Tykalová, Novotny, et al. (2021) in PD.

prosodic	phonatory-prosodic	articulatory-prosodic
monopitch	monopitch	monopitch
monoloudness	monoloudness	monoloudness
	reduced voice quality	
		articulatory deficits
female	male	male
	cognitive deficits	cognitive deficits
		axial symptoms

The idea of speech clusters is gaining attention again. A study by Rusz and colleagues postulates that clusters of speech types can be classified based on speech parameters, such as imprecise consonants (indicated by longer voice onset times in syllable repetitions of /pa-ta-ka/), harsh voice (indicated by cepstral peak prominence) and decreased voice quality (indicated by a lower harmonics-to-noise ratio), with the latter two being observed during sustained phonation of the vowel /a/ (Rusz, Tykalová, Novotny, et al., 2021). According to this study, three speech types can be defined that are presented in more detail in Table 4.1: prosodic, phonatory-prosodic, and articulatory-prosodic. The severity of speech impairment increases from the prosodic type to the phonatory-prosodic type and further to the articulatory-prosodic type, as more speech domains are affected throughout this process. This again highlights the development of speech deficits as a continuum from phonatory deficits, that appear first, to deficits affecting the articulation.

The study also investigated the response of levodopa therapy on speech in those three subtypes. Results indicate that only the phonatory-prosodic type benefits from levodopa therapy, leading to increased pitch modulation and improved voice quality (Rusz, Tykalová, Novotny, et al., 2021). The response may be based on the levodopa dosages, as they were highest in this speech type. In contrast, the articulatory-prosodic speech type did not respond to levodopa presumably because this type is characterized by the most severe motor impairment and more deficits in gait and posture. One can assume that axial symptoms are more related to articulatory deficits than to phonatory/prosodic ones. In line with this assumption, another study investigated the relationship between two alleged axial symptoms, freezing of gait and hypokinetic dysarthria, and comes to the conclusion that freezing is linked to articulatory features, such as vertical position of the tongue (jaw opening, measured with vowel formant F1), rather than phonatory-prosodic ones (Skodda et al., 2012).

It may be that the following causal chain applies: The greater the impairment in the axial domain, the more severe the freezing of gait and the more improper the articulation of tongue and jaw. In addition, Polychronis, Niccolini, Pagano, Yousaf, and Politis (2019) postulate that speech is more affected in patients of the akinetic-rigid subtype compared to those of the tremor-dominant type. Furthermore, Tykalová et al. (2020) describe that speech is more impaired in patients with postural instability and gait difficulties compared to the tremor-dominant type.

4.3 Treatment Effects on Speech

While treatments are effective for gross motor symptoms, it is yet to be fully understood how speech responds to levodopa treatment and STN-DBS. Reported results range from deterioration or improvement to no change at all. The next section will explore previous studies' ambiguous results about whether and how standard treatments affect speech production.

4.3.1 Effects of Levodopa

While levodopa is proven to be an effective treatment for gross motor performance (Katzenschlager & Lees, 2002), it remains unclear to what extent it influences speech production. Speech is classified as an axial symptom of PD and considered to be levodopa-resistant (Rascol et al., 2003). Therefore, speech changes due to levodopa intake are not necessarily expected.

To narrow down the selection of studies to be discussed, only studies whose methodology is based on a clear *levodopa challenge* (cf. Section 2.4.2) will be considered, since the drug dosage itself and the whole drug cycle may have an impact (De Letter et al., 2010). For this reason, only research is reported that compares medication-OFF condition (med-OFF; that is received after 12 hours of withdrawing PD medication) with medication-ON condition (med-ON; that is achieved with a controlled amount of levodopa given).

Previous acoustic studies investigated speech parameters in sustained vowel duration, a monologue or a reading task produced by parkinsonian speakers with moderate motor impairment in medication-OFF status, with UPDRS III scores ranging from 24 to 64. UPDRS III scores above 40 indicate an advanced PD development. All studies show agreement that motor impairment is improved under levodopa administration, but results on speech are inconsistent.

Heterogeneous results with respect to phonatory control are reported in the following. In 20 speakers with PD, an increased and more stable glottal control and a higher frequency of vocal fold movements were found in sustained phonation of the vowel /a/ (Sanabria et al., 2001). Cavallieri et al. (2021) report longer phonation times of the vowel /a/ only in female speakers. Noffs et al. (2017) observed no change in electromyographic patterns of the laryngeal muscles during vowel phonation in 19 speakers with PD. However, when investigating phonation in terms of pitch modulation related to prosodic marking, nuclear pitch contours were less deviant and more comparable to control speakers in 30 speakers with PD under levodopa (Frota et al., 2021). In a cohort representing late-stage PD, with a mean UPDRS III score of 64, no change in phonatory features was observed, although axial motor symptoms improved (Fabbri et al., 2017).

Azevedo et al. (2013) asked 10 speakers with PD to produce sentences in different modalities, such as certainty, doubt or declarative, and found that syllable durations were shorter under medication, while intensity and pitch values remained the same. In contrast, another study reports overall increased intensity values across all conditions, but also a greater extent of intensity decay over the time in nine English speakers with PD. The counting rate increased as well, while no changes with regard to pitch and articulation were found (Ho et al., 2008). With regard to reading in particular, Skodda, Grönheit, and Schlegel (2011) did not find changes in F0 variation and speech rate, but report that the typical decline during reading seemed to be counterbalanced by levodopa administration in this cohort of 20 speakers with PD.

De Letter, Santens, De Bodt, Boon, and Van Borsel (2006) determined no change in speech rate, but an increase of variability in 25 speakers with PD. On the other hand, a study on 15 speakers with PD performing a monologue and a reading task found slower speech rates under medication, but no change in intelligibility, naturalness, and voice quality (Spencer et al., 2009). Likewise, dysfluencies and verbal fluency seem to be unaffected by drug administration (Bayram et al., 2019; Im et al., 2019).

A study collection by Goberman and colleagues uniformly reports neither speech changes with regard to phonatory skills, speech and articulation rate nor to pause time and dysfluencies for nine speakers with PD when reading a text or producing a monologue, although motor impairment improved (Goberman et al., 2005; Goberman & Blomgren, 2003; Goberman et al., 2002). But it should be noted that in these studies levodopa administration was paused only for 8 hours prior to speech recordings.

The lacking effect of levodopa on speech parameters, such as intensity and pitch, that is often reported leads to the assumption that these speech domains do not correspond to the general motor network. In line with this, Elfmarková et al. (2016) demonstrated that the resting-state functional connectivity within brain networks that are related to prosody control does not change due to levodopa intake. Therefore, prosodic features might not be controlled in dopaminergic circuits.

When looking at vowel production, it seems that only some speakers with PD improve vowel articulation under levodopa. For five of 23 German speakers with PD, higher Vowel Articulation Indices could be measured for the vowels /i, a, u/, indicating an enhanced vowel space (Skodda et al., 2010). Okada, Murata, and Toda (2015) reported that the vowel space of 16 out of 21 Japanese speakers with PD was expanded under levodopa, without however reaching the size of control speakers. They analyzed five vowels comparable to peripheral vowels of German. In contrast, a more reduced and centralized vowel space was reported for 7 speakers with PD with regard to the vowels /i, a, u/ (Martel Sauvageau et al., 2015).

Only a few studies investigated underlying speech movements. An EMG study examined labial sounds in seven Swedish speakers with PD, while it should be noted that five of them underwent either unilateral or bilateral thalamotomy before. However, all speakers showed the same pattern regardless of thalamotomy, producing faster and smoother lip movements. These lead to an improved articulation of labial stops and an overall decrease of dysarthric symptoms (Leanderson et al., 1971). A more recent study analyzed lip movements and perioral stiffness in 10 speakers with PD producing syllable repetitions of /pa-pa-pa/ (Chu et al., 2015). They found greater perioral stiffness and increased lip amplitude under drug administration. The authors also detected a negative correlation between perioral stiffness and lower lip amplitude, noting that stiffness might be related to the overall rigidity that is present in PD (Chu et al., 2015). No changes in speech intelligibility and speech rate were found.

A study by Robertson et al. (2011) reported faster jaw movements in 27 speakers with PD under levodopa. Measurements were made with a kinesiograph. In line with these results, a study using electromagnetic articulography, found shorter, larger, and faster tongue movements in 16 speakers with PD producing vowels (Thies et al., 2021). As vocalic tongue movements were initiated later compared to medication-OFF condition, the movement planning seems to have been improved. However, the articulatory changes were not reflected in acoustic measures, as the Vowel Articulation Index and acoustic vowel duration did not change.

To summarize the articulatory results, the acoustic vowel space was observed to expand or remain the same under levodopa. The question arises to what extent axial symptoms affect the levodopa response and whether only those patients with less axial problems increase the vowel space under levodopa. Underlying speech movements are faster and larger after levodopa intake.

4.3.2 Effects of Deep Brain Stimulation

The following section will be focused on reviewing literature investigating the effects of bilateral STN-DBS on speech by mainly comparing conditions with activated (DBS-ON) and deactivated DBS (DBS-OFF). However, changes due to DBS implantation will be addressed as well.

In general, effects on speech due to STN-DBS are inconclusive in the literature, given that some speech skills improve, some remain the same and some worsen. In contrast, all previous studies are in agreement that STN-DBS improves motor functions significantly.

Implantation Effect

Results comparing the preoperative med-OFF status with the postoperative med-OFF/DBS-OFF condition will be summarized in this section, for the purpose of discussing the possible effect based of the mere presence of electrodes.

Comparing preoperative with postoperative speech output, lower intelligibility and therefore speech deterioration is described in 32 English-speaking patients with PD (Tripoliti et al., 2011). This could be reflected in longer, smaller or slower articulatory movements. Following on from this, Robertson et al. (2011) compared the speech of 14 patients with STN-DBS with that of 13 patients with GPi-DBS at baseline and six months after surgery. The STN-DBS group produced significantly slower jaw velocities, whereas this effect was not visible in the GPi-DBS group (Robertson et al., 2011). Similarly, Wang et al. (2006) found reduced articulatory precision after surgery comparing 20 English-speaking PD patients producing fast syllable repetitions of /pa-pa-pa, ta-ta-ta, ka-ka-ka/. Note that these patients had received only unilateral implants, with ten patients receiving DBS in the left STN and the other ten in the right STN. Another study reports no changes in syllable repetitions for Swedish-speaking patients with PD (Karlsson et al., 2011). In this context, a study highlights that high axial scores in the UPDRS III before surgery seem to be predictive for speech deterioration after implantation (Guehl et al., 2006).

DBS Effect

This section evaluates studies comparing deactivated and activated stimulation (DBS-OFF vs. DBS-ON) to find possible stimulation effects. As previous studies differ with regard to methodology, their results will be presented in two parts. In the first part, studies will be presented in which patients took their regular medication (med-ON). In part two studies are discussed in which drug administration was paused overnight (med-OFF).

MED-ON/DBS-OFF vs. *MED-ON/DBS-ON:* A study investigating intelligibility, articulation rate and F2 slopes in glides in a reading task did not report any changes for eight Quebec French-speaking patients with PD two to five years after DBS implantation (Martel-Sauvageau & Tjaden, 2017). However, during productions of monologues, higher speech rates were measured in 14 German-speaking patients in DBS-ON condition (Ehlen et al., 2020). An increased articulation rate with activated DBS was also determined by Karlsson et al. (2011). Seven Swedish-speaking patients with PD (two were unilaterally implanted in the left STN) increased the amount of syllables produced in fast syllable repetitions of /pa-pa-pa, ta-ta-ta, ka-ka-ka/. No change in articulation rate was found when repeating /pa-ta-ka/. Additionally, no change in the production of stop consonants was reported. In a follow-up study of the same research group, nine patients (two were unilaterally implanted in the left STN) performed a reading task 12 months after implantation. The analysis focused on stop consonant production and showed that under stimulation, the durations of frication in voiceless plosives were longer. The authors interpret this in terms of a more prominent acoustic release and therefore a more successful production of stop closures (Karlsson et al., 2014). Another study on Swedish-speaking patients assessed the ratings of articulatory precision from nine patients reading a text. No changes were indicated in a statistical analysis, but the authors mention a tendency towards reduced articulatory precision in DBS-ON condition (Eklund et al., 2015). However, articulatory precision was clearly reduced in comparison to recordings in med-ON condition before implantation.

With regard to vowel articulation, one study compared intelligibility and naturalness ratings as well as the vowel space area of 56 Japanese-speaking patients with PD with deactivated and activated DBS (Tanaka et al., 2016). Vowel formant frequencies of /i, a, u/ were obtained during sustained vowel phonation and included in order to measure the vowel space. The vowel space area was larger in DBS-ON condition, whereas perceptual ratings did not differ between the two conditions. In DBS-OFF the values of the ratio indicating the vowel space area strongly correlated with reduced intelligibility and naturalness. In addition, a small study recorded target words with CVCV structure embedded in a carrier sentence. The target words consisted of the same three vowels and alternating consonants (Martel Sauvageau et al., 2014). For eight Quebec French-speaking patients the authors reported a larger and less centralized vowel space under stimulation but no change in vocalic segment duration. The different consonants influenced vowel articulation to the same extent in DBS-OFF and DBS-ON condition.

Studies on phonatory-glottal control found increased intensity values during fast syllable repetitions with activated DBS in eight Swedish-speaking individuals 12 months after surgery (Lundgren et al., 2011). However, a study by Tanaka et al. (2015), conducted with 68 Japanese-speaking patients, reports that 60 % of the patients produced more voiceless speech portions under activated DBS, indicating a reduced glottal control. These deficits were more often present in females and did not improve with deactivated DBS.

A study by (Dromey & Bjarnason, 2011) highlights the variability in speech patterns across patients. They investigated speech in six English-speaking patients with PD, reporting that intelligibility ratings and verbal fluency reduce under stimulation, while results for glottal control and articulation are variable. Glottal control improved and worsened in half of the patients respectively. Moreover, four out of six patients had smaller vowel space areas in DBS-ON condition.

Regular drug administration is very individual and drug doses differ across patients, which makes it difficult to derive the DBS effect adequately from the results summarized above. The next section will take a look at studies aiming to capture the pure effect of DBS independent of individual drug administration by assuming that patients are stimulated under the optimal stimulation settings for perfect motor control.

MED-OFF/DBS-OFF vs. MED-OFF/DBS-ON: Two studies compared the speech of up to seven English-speaking patients with PD in repetition and conversation tasks in both stimulation conditions (Sidtis & Sidtis, 2017; van Lancker Sidtis et al., 2010). In the repetition task higher harmonics-to-noise ratios in DBS-ON were reported, indicating an improved voice quality. Besides improved glottal control, patients exhibited less intelligible and less fluent speech in DBS-ON condition, especially in spontaneous speech. Improved voice quality with activated DBS was also reported by Skodda et al. (2014) based on perceptual ratings of the speech output of 38 German-speaking patients. They noted a trend towards an additionally improved prosodic function by means of increased intensity and pitch variability. Eight out of these 38 patients had an overall more severe speech impairment and pronounced articulatory deficits.

Fast syllable repetitions, such as /pa-pa-pa, ta-ta-ta, ka-ka-ka/, produced by 20 English-speaking patients with PD were rated as less precise with regard to articulatory precision (Wang et al., 2006). Note that these patients received unilateral STN-DBS; ten patients were unilaterally implanted in the left STN and ten in the right STN. As unilateral DBS implantation is not common in patients with PD, these results might not reflect patterns that can be observed elsewhere, and especially unilateral stimulation in the left STN can worsen speech, as will be described below.

A small study observed shorter and more frequent pauses in spontaneous speech of seven English-speaking patients in DBS-ON condition (Ahn et al., 2014). Shorter pauses were also found by Gentil, Pinto, Pollak, and Benabid (2003), who investigated sentence production in 16 French-speaking individuals with PD. They also recorded sustained vowel durations and fast syllable repetitions. Patients presented longer maximum phonation times, a more stable voice, and higher repetition rates but no changes in intensity values under stimulation.

Acoustic measurements of vowels were made by Sidtis, Alken, Tagliati, Alterman, and van Lancker Sidtis (2016). Seven English-speaking males produced sustained vowel phonation of the vowels /i, a, u/. The vowel space area was calculated at two points: Shortly after the beginning and around the midpoint of each production. It was larger at the beginning in DBS-OFF compared to DBS-ON condition. But the values declined towards the midpoint in DBS-OFF. While this decline was also present in the control group, it was not in DBS-ON. The values remained stable but overall smaller, indicating a reduced vowel space and changes in speech initiation or planning. In general, more changes were found in the vowel frequencies of the vowels /i/ and /a/ compared to /u/.

There are a few studies that analyzed the compression forces of articulators, such as the upper lip, the lower lip, and the tongue, in speakers of French. An early study reports reduced forces when comparing DBS-OFF and DBS-ON condition in ten patients exhibiting less precise movements, articulatory undershoot and later initiation of tongue movements in DBS-OFF condition. Variability was also higher in DBS-OFF condition. However, in DBS-ON condition patients achieved the same force level as healthy controls (Gentil et al., 1999). A follow-up study from 2003 presented the same results for 16 patients (Gentil et al., 2003). Articulatory forces increased with activated DBS and movements were more precise. The strongest were found at the lower lip (by about 93 %), followed by the upper lip (74 %) and the tongue (66 %). A similar amount of force gain was reported by Pinto, Gentil, Fraix, Benabid, and Pollak (2003) for 26 French-speaking individuals, confirming the beneficial effect of STN-DBS on articulators (84 % lower lip, 52 % upper lip, 68 % tongue).

To sum up, activated DBS can lead to improved voice function, higher breath support, and more precise articulatory movements. The articulatory precision is not reflected on the acoustic level because a trend towards smaller acoustic vowel spaces is reported. However, the vowel space can become larger again under levodopa.

A few studies performed more complex investigations by comparing at least four conditions, changing not only the stimulation condition, but also the medication status. These studies captured the interaction between DBS and drug administration (Martel Sauvageau et al., 2015; Hartinger et al., 2011). The results are difficult to interpret due to small sample sizes and different investigated speech domains. As expected for small sample sizes, variable results were reported in a study investigating four French-speaking patients three to five years after surgery (Pinto et al., 2005), as well as in a study on two German-speaking patients (Hartinger et al., 2011). Another study on 12 Italian-speaking patients reported no deterioration of speech due to DBS, improvement in voice features, such as voice tremor and overall glottal control, and found the DBS effect to be more beneficial than the one of levodopa (D'Alatri et al., 2008). No differences in acoustic measures of sustained vowel phonation, sentence production, and syllable repetitions of /pa-ta-ka/ were determined in 11 Chinese-speaking individuals by Xie et al. (2011). However, the authors highlight that only female speakers changed their articulation of the vowel /i/, indicating that this vowel might be more sensitive to improvement with DBS.

Stimulation Settings and Electrode Position

The treatments of patients with PD are as heterogeneous as the symptoms that can occur. Therefore, the individual therapy should be taken into account, since medication doses, electrode locations, and DBS settings may differ and thus lead to different effects on speech (Martel Sauvageau et al., 2015).

A deterioration of speech after or during DBS, is referred to as *stimulation-induced dysarthria*. To avoid this side effect, low-frequency DBS (at around 60 to 80 Hz) is favored, as it was found to lead to improved intelligibility and acoustic vowel expansion (Phokaewvarangkul et al., 2019; Knowles et al., 2018; Åström et al., 2010). In contrast, high-frequency stimulation around 130 Hz leads to lower intensity values and reduced articulatory and phonatory control (Morello et al., 2020; Phokaewvarangkul et al., 2019). In a review, Fox et al. (2012) note moreover that loud speech cues are reduced in individuals with high-frequency DBS.

Besides stimulation frequency, other parameters that impact speech after DBS implantation are the micro lesion effect, electrode position, voltage, and the stimulated brain tissue around the activated contact. Regarding electrode position, electrodes positioned outside the STN can worsen speech (Pinto et al., 2005). Moreover, electrodes positioned medial and/or posterior to the center of the subthalamic nucleus were recognized as having a potentially negative effect (Åström et al., 2010), as posterior electrode locations were associated with a worsening of speech production (Jorge et al., 2020). The same is valid for activated contacts. Speech improves when active contacts lie inside or in the superior part of the STN, but worsens if they are located in the postereolateral part (Tripoliti et al., 2011). Lower intensity values were reported when active contacts were positioned in the dorsal zone rather than the ventral zone (Phokaewvarangkul et al., 2019).

Unilateral stimulation can also impact speech. It has been shown that speech is negatively affected in the domain of prosody when only contacts in the left STN are activated (Santens et al., 2003). Especially amplitude and voltage are responsible for this impact (Tripoliti et al., 2011). Also, articulatory precision and speech rate are reported to be reduced under unilateral left STN stimulation (Wang et al., 2006). Note that most of the patients with PD have bilateral DBS and that it is rather uncommon to only activate the stimulation in the left STN.

In addition, when stimulation involves the dentatorubrothalamic tract, speech deteriorates at least for patients of the akinetic-rigid subtype (Fenoy et al., 2016). The dentatorubrothalamic tract is a fiber tract that connects the cerebellum to the thalamus.

4.3.3 Levodopa vs DBS

This section focuses on treatment by comparing speech in a group treated only medically with a group treated with DBS. The comparison will therefore be, med-ON vs. DBS-ON. According to Tsuboi et al. (2015), STN-DBS reduces intelligibility in most patients, whereas voice tremor or monoloudness improves compared to the medically treated group. Another study compared two groups, one medical group and one DBS group with 8 patients each, at baseline and after one year. This study reported no change in intelligibility, but higher sound pressure in sustained phonation in the group receiving DBS compared to a group in their best medical treatment condition (Tripoliti et al., 2006).

In contrast, studies with large sample sizes report higher voice impairment and reduced intensity values under DBS. One study compared 50 Thai-speaking patients with PD treated with medication to 50 patients that were treated with DBS. The DBS group had undergone DBS implantation four years prior to the speech assessment (Phokaewvarangkul et al., 2019). Results indicate that the DBS group has higher voice impairment, assessed with the Voice Handicap Index, and lower intensities. Voice quality was also lower in 68 Japanese-speaking patients with STN-DBS compared to 40 medically-treated patients (Tanaka et al., 2015).

A study by Tanaka et al. (2016) investigated the speech of 56 Japanese-speaking patients with DBS and 41 medically-treated patients. Perceptual ratings indicated reduced intelligibility and naturalness in the DBS group. Reasons for the low ratings were, for example, imprecise consonant production and variation in speech rate, among other parameters. Vowel frequencies of the vowels /i, a, u/ were taken to measure the vowel space area. While there were no differences in the vowel space area between the medically-treated group and the DBS group with deactivated DBS, the vowel space area was larger with activated DBS compared to the medically-treated group. Moreover, Tanaka et al. (2021) report higher rate instability in a DBS group of 26 patients that was compared to a medically-treated group of 44 patients producing syllable repetitions of /pa-pa-pa/.

These comparisons call into question whether DBS is superior to drug treatment regarding speech. Moreover, all findings reported in this chapter further highlight the importance to differentiate dysarthric speech as a symptom of PD from dysarthric speech as side effect of a treatment, such as dopaminergic therapy or DBS. Therefore, disease-related and treatment-related changes need to be disentangled.

To conclude, not only levodopa treatment but also STN-DBS improves motor impairment in PD. But with regard to speech and taking into account the heterogeneous results, the question remains why it is that motor symptoms improve, but speech responds differently to treatment. Since symptoms in PD manifest and progress in different ways in each individual, the observed patterns are particularly heterogeneous in nature (Delvaux et al., 2018). Moreover, Pinto et al. (2005) point out that all patients react differently, regarding both improvement and exacerbation. This has to be kept in mind when studying speech in PD.

4.4 Research Questions

The study of speech motor functions has established itself as an exciting and important field of research. Many acoustic studies have been carried out that gave a detailed account of speech changes in terms of pitch and loudness modulation, investigating the clearly reduced and centralized articulation space as well as the less intelligible speech output in speakers with PD.

However, there is relatively little research on changes in the underlying articulatory movements on the one hand, and only a small amount of data on treatment effects on speech movements on the other hand. Whereas differences between healthy control speakers and speakers with PD are well elaborated, the effects of standard treatments on speech are inconclusive. And while treatment effects for gross motor symptoms are clearly visible, it is still not well understood how speech responds to levodopa treatment and STN-DBS.

Moreover, a description of what takes place under the acoustic surface is still missing. Therefore, the aim of this work is to contribute to the sparse literature by shedding light on the underlying speech movements of the tongue body producing vocalic sounds. Electromagnetic articulography allows speech movements to be examined directly to understand the articulatory mechanisms that lead to reduced and increased speech intelligibility. Such knowledge is critical for improving the clinical management of speech disturbances in individuals with PD.

This dissertation will add data to the existing research by comparing articulatory speech patterns in healthy controls and speakers with PD. On the other hand, this patient cohort was looked at for the first time with electromagnetic articulography pre-surgery and post-surgery to investigate the effects of standard treatment methods patients have to deal with during the course of PD. The data of individuals with PD will be compared across four conditions to capture the treatment effects: medication-OFF, medication-ON, medication-OFF with activated DBS, and medication-OFF with deactivated DBS.

As it has been elaborated in this chapter, especially speed, range, precision and timing patterns of articulatory movements are of importance when investigating speech in PD. Therefore, this dissertation focuses on spatio-temporal features of tongue body movements during vowel production, since vocalic movements are poorly studied, and covers the following questions:

Production - Kinematics:

- Do speakers with PD differ in tongue movement range and speed from healthy control speakers?
- Do timing patterns of vocalic onsets and targets differ between speakers with PD and healthy controls?
- Are speakers with PD able to adjust articulatory speech pattern (e.g. in the context of prosodic marking)?

Perception - Intelligibility:

- Do reduced tongue movement ranges result in less intelligible speech?

- Does greater gross motor impairment correlate with reduced intelligibility?

Gross Motor Status - Impairment and Treatment Effects:

- Is articulatory impairment related to axial motor deficits?
- Do articulatory patterns in speakers with PD change with drug and/or surgical treatment?
- Is drug treatment superior to surgical treatment with regard to speech?

The methodological approach of this work will be presented in the following chapter. More detailed research questions are formulated at the beginning of each result chapter so that the relevant hypotheses are given per analysis.

5 Methods

5.1 Objectives

The aim of this study is to investigate the speech of patients with Parkinson's disease (PD) and to determine the changes that occur on the articulatory level due to the disease, levodopa intake, and deep brain stimulation. The main focus lies on articulatory movements of the tongue body during vowel production. One speech task in which adjustments of articulatory features are commonly observed is prosodic prominence marking. Please note that in this study the elicitation of prominence marking is not used to further the understanding of the encoding of prosodic structures. It will rather be used to capture strategies of prominence marking in PD involving adjustments of speech parameters in the spatial and temporal domain on the articulatory level. Depending on the degree of prosodic prominence, articulatory changes differ within the relevant speech unit, as speech effort is enhanced or reduced (cf. Section 3.3.2). This allows articulatory movement patterns to be investigated in more detail. Therefore, the experiment is designed to examine how articulators perform in PD on a continuum under varying speech demands. The exact experimental implementation, the subjects involved, the speech material, and the measurements are described in detail in the following sections.

5.2 Participants

13 patients[2] with idiopathic Parkinson's disease (9 male, 4 female) aged between 42 and 70 years and 13 age- and sex-matched healthy controls participated in the study (Table 5.1). The study was approved by the local ethics committee of the University of Cologne (18–425; date of approval

---

2   Originally, 17 patients were included in the study. But due to the Coronavirus disease (COVID-19) pandemic that began in 2019, 4 out of 17 patients did not show up to the second appointment. The sample size is still comparable to previous research conducting articulatory recordings with patients in two treatment conditions (cf. Mücke et al., 2018).

was February 8, 2019). All participants gave a written informed consent before participating in the study.

Table 5.1. Demographics of patients with PD and age- and sex-matched healthy controls.

Patients	Sex	Age	Controls	Sex	Age
PD01	m	69	CON01	m	69
PD02	f	51	CON02	f	48
PD03	m	63	CON03	m	62
PD04	m	54	CON04	m	55
PD05	m	68	CON05	m	67
PD06	m	56	CON06	m	57
PD07	f	70	CON07	f	71
PD08	m	53	CON08	m	53
PD09	f	69	CON09	f	67
PD10	m	42	CON10	m	45
PD11	m	59	CON11	m	58
PD12	m	56	CON12	m	57
PD13	f	56	CON13	f	59

The main inclusion criteria for all participants was that they had to be native speakers of German. Exclusion criteria were the presence of dementia and/or depression, preexisting neurological conditions like a stroke or a history of previously induced speech problems. A potential presence of dementia was assessed with the use of the *Parkinson Neuropsychometric Dementia Assessment* (PANDA). The PANDA is a screening tool consisting of different cognitive tasks assessing the learning and memory function, verbal fluency, visuospatial functions, and working memory. Values below 14 indicate symptoms of dementia (Kalbe et al., 2008). In addition, the *mini-mental state examination* (MMSE, cut-off < 19) was applied as an established clinical tool for the diagnosis of dementia. It has been reported in a number of previous studies (Kukull et al., 1994; Folstein et al., 1975). Depressive symptoms were operationalized with the *Beck-Depression-Inventory-II* (BDI-II) which is a 21-item self-report questionnaire asking participants to respond to questions regarding changes in, e.g. mood and feelings, motivation and pleasure, suicidality, sleep and energy, and weight, among other things within the previous two weeks. Values below 14 indicate no or minimal symptoms of depression

(Beck et al., 1996). Moreover, participants who were allergic to latex could not participate since latex was used in the experimental speech recording sessions.

Patients with PD were included in the study if they were clinically diagnosed with the idiopathic Parkinson syndrome according to the Brain Bank criteria of the United Kingdom Parkinson's disease society (Hughes et al., 1992). Assessment by a speech therapist with expertise in neurogenic speech disorders excluded the presence of other speech and language problems, such as aphasia, apraxia of speech, or developmental speech disorders. All patients had only mild dysarthric symptoms based on their conglomerated performance in a reading task, spontaneous speech, maximum vowel phonation, oral diadochokinesis and modulation of loudness and pitch. None of the patients reported difficulties with swallowing. No restrictions were applied to disease duration or severity of dysarthria in order to investigate the impact of disease severity on the observed speech patterns. Patients were only treated with medication prior to study inclusion. Nevertheless, all patients were interested in alternative treatment methods, such as a DBS, because the drugs they had been taking had a reduced and/or shorter effect, and/or they had already experienced motor fluctuations (cf. Section 2.3.1). All patients were recruited during an in-hospital stay and were visited twice over a period of time, once before the implantation of DBS and a second time 5 to 13 months after surgery[3].

5.3 Data Elicitation

The study was conducted at the Department of Neurology of the University Hospital in Cologne. As described above, all participants completed a neuropsychological assessment beforehand to exclude cognitive impairment or depression - two factors that could have an impact on the subjects' speech performance.

In addition, the participants' motor functions and speech performance were tested. Motor functions were determined according to part III of the

---

3 The plan was to test all patients after 6 months, but due to the Coronavirus disease (COVID-19) pandemic since 2019, some re-test appointments had to be rescheduled or postponed.

UPDRS (Fahn et al., 1987), as described in section 2.4.1. The motor functions of the control group were assessed with the same scale to take into account age effects on motor skills. Each motor assessment was videotaped, to allow the ratings to be performed later by a qualified neurologist who is proficient and was blind to group and treatment condition. Values of the total rating score will be reported further down together with several subscores for rigidity, bradykinesia, axial symptoms as well as postural instability and gait difficulties (PIGD) (cf. Rusz, Cmejla, Růžička, et al., 2013). Higher values indicate a more severe motor impairment.

The speech recording process is explained in more detail under section 5.4. In order to obtain a subjective assessment of the speaking ability of the subjects themselves, each participant was asked to classify their ability to speak on a 10 cm visual analog scale (VAS). Higher values indicate a better speaking ability (0 cm indicates the lowest speaking ability and 10 cm the highest). These values help to assess whether the participants (patients in particular) evaluate their speech in the same way as professionals or whether the perception differs.

The healthy controls participated once in the study, while the subjects from the PD group took part twice. Patients with PD were assessed i) before the implantation of STN-DBS and ii) 5 to 13 months after the implantation. The second assessment after this period minimizes possible confounding effects due to disease progression (Cersosimo et al., 2009) and ensures that the DBS effect is stabilized. Per visit, preoperative as well as postoperative, patients were examined in two conditions, which will be explained in the following subsections 5.3.1 and 5.3.2. Therefore, each patient with PD completed the motor assessment and additionally took part in the speech recordings in a total of four conditions (preoperative in medication-OFF and medication-ON, and postoperative with deactivated and activated DBS). In addition, the levodopa equivalent daily dose of each patient was calculated based on their current medication plan at both visits, as dosages may differ from the preoperative visit (Tomlinson et al., 2010).

Hence, the components of the experiment included the UPDRS III motor assessment according to its guidelines, the rating on the VAS, and the speech recordings. The healthy control participants performed these parts of the experiment in a randomized order. Randomization options for the patient recordings were limited, as will be explained below.

5.3.1 Preoperative Assessment

Patients with PD were first assessed before the implantation of STN-DBS. These preoperative recordings were conducted in the following two conditions: i) medication-OFF (med-OFF) and ii) medication-ON (med-ON). The OFF-state is defined as abstinence of at least 12 hours from PD medication, such as levodopa. To guarantee abstinence over this period of time prior to recording, the patients' evening medication (after 6 pm) the day before the recording as well as the morning medication on the day of the assessment were left off. For logistical reasons, the preoperative recordings started in med-OFF condition, when the drugs were not in effect.

The morning of the first trial day started with the recording of the UPDRS III video, followed by the subjective evaluation of the patients' speech performance on the VAS in med-OFF condition. Thereafter, the speech recordings were made. Before a short break, patients received 200 mg of soluble *Madopar LT* (100/25 mg Levodopa + Benserazid). 30 to 40 minutes after drug intake, the second UPDRS III video was taken followed by the second speech recording. Afterwards, the VAS was rated in med-ON condition by the participants (Table 5.2).

Table 5.2. Procedure preoperative recording sessions.

time	task	condition
08.30 - 08.45 am	UPDRS III video	
08.45 - 08.50 am	VAS rating	med-OFF
08.50 - 09.30 am	Speech recording	
09.30 - 10.15 am	*200mg levodopa intake and break*	
10.15 - 10.30 am	UPDRS III video	
10.30 - 10.55 am	Speech recording	med-ON
10.55 - 11.00 am	VAS rating	

5.3.2 Postoperative Assessment

Postoperative recordings were scheduled 5 to 13 months after the implantation of the neurostimulator and accompanied by a follow-up examination in hospital. Electrodes of all patients were implanted in the dorso-lateral STN in each hemisphere, as Figure 5.1 shows.

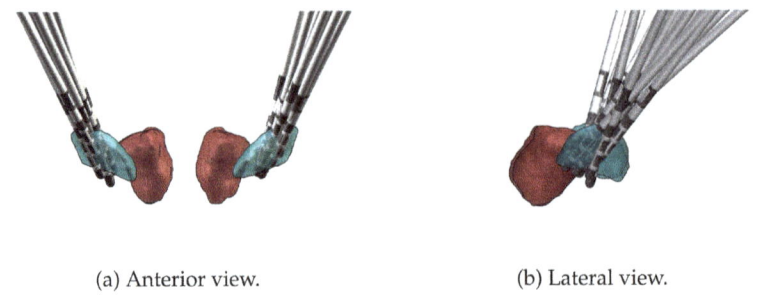

(a) Anterior view.   (b) Lateral View.

Figure 5.1. Lead electrodes of all patients. Electrode tips are located within the dorso-lateral subthalamic nucleus (blue). Contact positions are shown in relation the nucleus ruber (red).

As in the case of the preoperative recordings, PD medication was again suspended for at least 12 hours before the recording. However, the neurostimulation remained activated overnight in the regular stimulation setting. In contrast to the preoperative recordings, the sequence of the stimulation condition was randomized, so that half of the patients were recorded first with deactivated stimulation (DBS-OFF) and then with activated stimulation (DBS-ON), while the other half was recorded in the opposite order (Table 5.3).

Table 5.3. Procedure postoperative recording sessions.

time	task	condition
08.30 - 08.45 am	UPDRS III video	
08.45 - 08.50 am	VAS rating	DBS-ON or DBS-OFF
08.50 - 09.30 am	Speech recording	
09.30 - 10.00 am	*Switching DBS OFF/ON and break*	
10.00 - 10.15 am	UPDRS III video	
10.15 - 10.45 am	Speech recording	DBS-OFF or DBS-ON
10.45 - 11.00 am	VAS rating	

The session started with the recording of the UPDRS III video, followed by the subjective evaluation of the patients' speech performance rating on the VAS. Thereafter, the speech recordings were made. Before a break of 30 minutes, the neurostimulator was turned OFF or ON respectively. Patients in DBS-ON condition were tested under their regular stimulation settings. These settings are listed in the appendix A.1. After the break, the second UPDRS III video was taken, followed by the speech recording and another VAS rating.

5.4 Speech Recordings

5.4.1 Set-up

The experimental set up was the same across participants and recording conditions. All speech recordings took place in a quiet room with sound-absorbing partition walls at the Department of Neurology of the University Hospital in Cologne. Speech data were recorded acoustically and kinematically. The acoustic signal was captured using a condenser microphone headset (AKG C 544 L) keeping a constant mouth-to-microphone distance of about 7 cm throughout the recording session. The acoustic signal was recorded at 44.1 kHz/16 bit. The gain level was adjusted between the recording sessions and conditions. Therefore, a reference tone (pure tone, 440 Hz) was recorded as the first stimulus of each recording based on which the intensity levels of the audios for the perception experiment were controlled.

The kinematic data were recorded using a 3D Electromagnetic Articulograph (EMA, Carstens Medizinelektronik GmbH, AG 501 Twin). Prior to the experimental session, sensors were coated with latex for protection, but also to slightly increase the adhesive surface. Six sensors were placed in the head region of each subject by using tissue adhesive, a non-toxic glue: (1) left ear, (2) right ear, (3) lower lip, (4) upper lip, (5) tongue body, and (6) tongue tip. Sensors 1 and 2 function as reference points for correcting head movements, while sensors 3 to 6 track the active articulators. Tongue sensors were placed approximately 1 cm (tongue tip) and 4 cm (tongue body) from the tip of the tongue.

As patients were given a break between the two conditions (OFF and ON), sometimes the sensors on the tongue were detached or fell off. To guarantee that the sensors were placed in the same positions in all four recording conditions, photos of the tongue with the sensors were taken in the very first condition (med-OFF). Moreover, color-coded circles were drawn around the sensors with food dye to mark their exact positions within each session. This made it easier to place the sensors in the same spot in the postoperative recordings or in case they fell off.

The speech recordings consisted of three different tasks performed in a randomized order across speakers and recording conditions: (1) oral diadochokinesis, (2) prominence production, and (3) sentence production. In this dissertation, however, only the results on prosodic prominence marking will be discussed in more detail.

5.4.2 Speech Task and Speech Material

As already described in section 3.3, the speech system is flexible and typically adjusts to (task-)specific demands. A speech task was chosen to elicit adjustments of specific articulatory speech parameters in the temporal and spatial domain. The purpose of this work is to examine the extent to which patients with PD make use of the strategies of prominence marking and whether their modificational abilities are limited by the disorder or treatment methods.

The selection of speech material presents itself as challenging. Applying a more controlled setting, such as a reading text, provides the most comparable speech units, but at the same time speech production is less naturalistic. To investigate speech resembling daily life communication, a conversation seems to be the more adequate choice, however it allows for little control over speech units (Kent et al., 1999). In an attempt to find a balance between these two options, a speech task was designed as a question-answer-scenario to elicit more natural speech production, while also maintaining control over the speech material. The target words were disyllabic female names ($C_1V_1.C_2V_2$-structure) with word stress on the first syllable (Figure 5.2).

- C1 was either a labial or alveolar sound: /m, l/
- V1 was one of the five German peripheral vowels: /i, e, a, o, u/
- C2 was an alveolar sound: /l/ if C1 is labial; /n/ if C1 is alveolar
- V2 was either /i/ or /ɐ/

The target words were embedded in a predefined sentence structure, which differed in the subject (Opa, *grandpa*; Oma, *grandma*; Schwester, *sister*; Bruder, *brother*) and the verb (gewunken, *waved*; verlassen, *left*), such as:

- Der Opa hat der Mila gewunken. *(The grandpa waved at Mila.)*
- Die Schwester hat die Mali verlassen. *(The sister left Mali.)*

Note that it is rather uncommon for standard German to have an article before a name. The article was used to control underlying articulatory movements to be able to track their trajectories. It is easier to distinguish individual movements from each other when visible changes appear before and after. By using articles, open and closed vowels were alternated in adjacent position to the target syllable. This means that if the target word ended with an /a/, the preceding article was /deɐ/. If the target word ended with an /i/, the preceding article was /di:/. This allowed the movements of the tongue back to be investigated in the best possible way. Moreover, as all five peripheral vowels were included, it was possible to analyze the whole vowel space and all tongue body positions in the horizontal domain (from front to back) and in the vertical domain (from raised to lowered). And since, the consonant C1 varied regarding the place of articulation, the data also allowed for movements of the lower lip (/m/) and the tongue tip (/l/) to be analyzed. However, the focus of this work will be on vowel production.

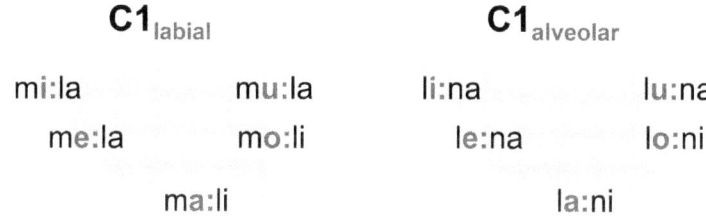

C1$_{labial}$		C1$_{alveolar}$	
mi:la	mu:la	li:na	lu:na
me:la	mo:li	le:na	lo:ni
	ma:li		la:ni

Figure 5.2. Ten target words grouped by the place of articulation of the first consonant C1.

In order to elicit speech that is as spontaneous and natural as possible, a game-like application was programmed. This application was presented on a TV screen. Depending on the carrier sentence, the participant watched a scene in which a person (grandma, grandpa, sister, brother) either leaves the room ('leaving' - scene) or comes into the room and waves ('waving'-scene). In both scenes a girl introduced with her name is sitting on a chair. Each scene consisted of three parts, as depicted in Figure 5.3a. The scenes were animated so that the actions of waving, leaving or speaking were visible in the video.

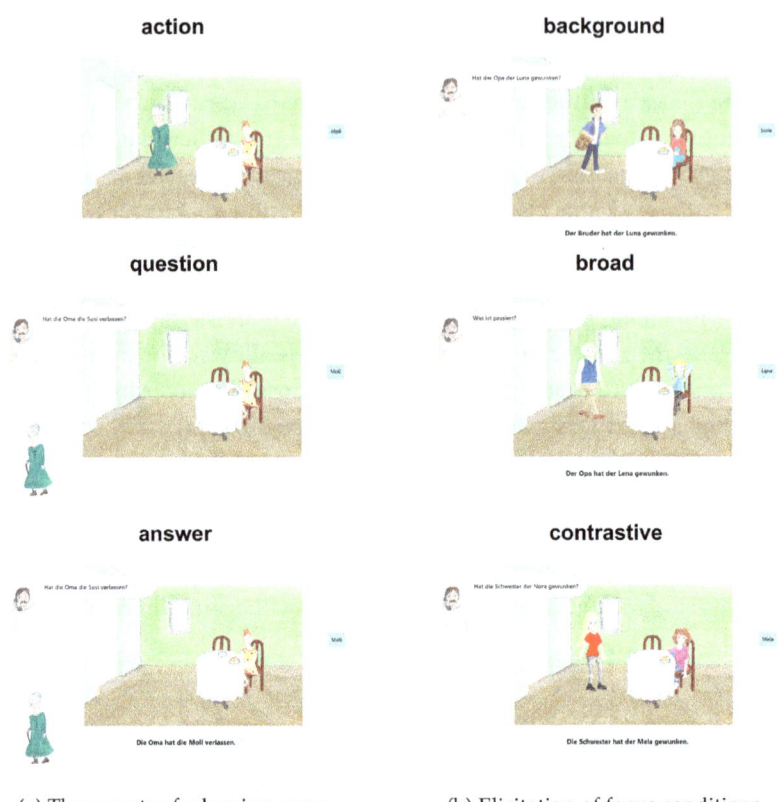

(a) Three parts of a leaving-scene.   (b) Elicitation of focus conditions.

Figure 5.3. Procedure of data elicitation using a question-answer-scenario.

1. **Action:** A person either enters the room and waves, or leaves the room.
2. **Question:** After the person finishes their action of leaving or waving, the father of the girl appears and asks a question to the participant. The question is presented visually and auditorily.
3. **Answer:** The participant is instructed to answer the question in the given sentence structure. In case assistance is needed, the correct answer sentence is displayed a few seconds after the question was asked. The participants are allowed to respond before the answer is shown.

The target words appeared in three different focus structures: background, broad focus, and contrastive focus (cf. Section 3.3.2). To elicit the target words in these three focus conditions, various scenarios were created (Figure 5.3b, Table 5.4). To elicit the target word in background condition, the name of the girl in the question corresponded to the name of the girl sitting on the chair. In this case, there is a contrast between the person in action (brother) and the person the father is asking about (grandpa), so that the girl's name is in the background (cf. Table 5.4 for background condition, grandpa vs. brother). Conversely, in the scenario eliciting the target word in contrastive focus condition, the father gets the name of the person in action right (sister), but not the name of the girl who is being waved at, putting her name (Mela) in contrastive focus (cf. Table 5.4 for contrastive focus, Nora vs. Mela). In the broad focus context, the father asks an open question about what happens in the scene, so that the entire answer contains new information that is of interest to him (cf. Table 5.4 for broad focus).

Table 5.4. Examples of question-answer-scenarios to elicit target words in three different focus conditions: background, broad focus, and contrastive focus.

Background (girl's name is already given, not accented)	
Bruder tritt ein und winkt.	*(The brother enters and waves.)*
Hat der Opa der Luna gewunken?	(Was grandpa waving to Luna?)
Der **Bruder** hat der Luna gewunken.	(The **brother** was waving to Luna.)
Broad focus (girl's name is new, accented)	
Opa tritt ein und winkt.	*(The grandpa enters and waves.)*
Was ist passiert?	(What happened?)
Der **Opa** hat der **Lena** gewunken.	(The **grandpa** was waving to **Lena**.)
Contrastive focus (girl's name is new and name corrected, accented)	
Schwester tritt ein und winkt.	*(The sister enters and waves.)*
Hat die Schwester der Nora gewunken?	(Was the sister waving to Nora?)
Die Schwester hat der **Mela** gewunken.	(The sister was waving to **Mela**.)

With regard to prominence marking, the broad focus condition will be taken as the starting point, as it represents a more neutral condition. For comparison, the elicitation of background and contrastive focus productions were included to investigate whether speakers with PD can actively and consciously reduce articulatory effort for the background condition on the one hand, and strongly modulate articulatory parameters, on the other hand, to increase the functional load for the contrastive focus condition. This set-up makes it possible to test the ability and the flexibility of the speech system in PD.

A test phase was included at the beginning of the speech task. During this phase, all target words (female names) were produced in isolation. Three test trials were carried out to provide participants with the opportunity to familiarize not only with uncommon names and the task itself, but also with speaking with sensors attached. No filler items were used and no repetitions were made in order not to prolong the duration of the experiment in consideration of the patients' condition. Only utterances that were produced incorrectly were repeated. In total, 1950 items were recorded:

- 13 speakers with PD x 4 treatment conditions x 10 target words x 3 focus conditions
- 13 healthy control speakers x 1 condition x 10 target words x 3 focus conditions

In the end, 1928 items went into the final acoustic analysis and 1916 items went into the final articulatory analysis, as some productions were excluded due to mispronunciation or sensor tracking errors. Note that one speaker with PD (PD03) did not tolerate the DBS-OFF condition so that he did not perform the experiment in this condition.

5.5 Speech Data Processing

The kinematic data were corrected for head movements using the software provided by Carstens Medizinelektronik GmbH. After head correction, the kinematic data were converted into ssff-format to be displayed and further processed in the EMU-webAPP of the EMU-SDMS environment (Winkelmann et al., 2017). As the data analysis focuses on the midsagittal plane, only the y-axis (showing the raising and lowering of the tracked articulator) and the x-axis (indicating the fronting and retracting) were displayed[4].

---

4   The 3-dimensional kinematic data displays movements on the x-axis, the y-axis, and on the z-axis. Regularly, movements along the x-axis represent fronting or retraction of the tracked articulator, the y-axis represents movements to the left or right side, and the z-axis indicates a raising or lowering of the articulator. Note, that in this work the orientation of the y- and z- axes are swapped by the converter.

After the data were manually annotated according to the guidelines explained below, they were extracted using the packages *emuR* (Winkelmann et al., 2021) and *praatR* (Albin, 2014) in R (R Core Team, 2022).

5.5.1 Annotation

Acoustics

On the acoustic level, target words, stressed syllables, and their respective segments were annotated according to the speech waveform and the wideband spectrogram. Inspection of higher formant structures was used to especially identify segmental boundaries between consonantal sounds and vowels, as higher formant structures are considerably reduced in laterals and nasals, such as /m/ and /l/ (Ladefoged & Johnson, 2014). The nasals were additionally identified by antiformants. As the main domain of prominence production in German is the stressed syllable, the first syllable of the target words ($C_1 V_1$) is of interest for this data set.

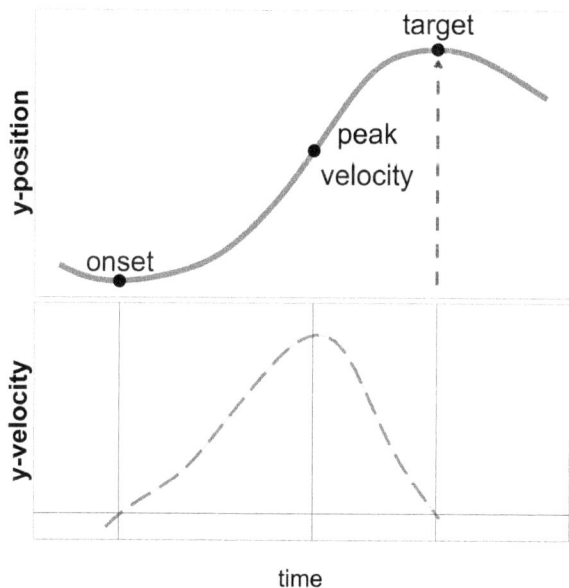

Figure 5.4. Annotation of three articulatory landmarks. Onset and target are identified by zero-crossings in the velocity trace. Peak velocity is aligned with the maximum in the velocity trace.

Articulatory Movements

The annotation of articulatory movements was focused on the movements involved in the production of the sounds in the first stressed syllable. Therefore, the movements of the lower lip, the tongue tip, and the tongue body within the stressed syllable (C_1V_1) were annotated. Articulatory movements for the production of C1 were annotated on the movement trajectory of either the lower lip (for production of the bilabial nasal /m/) or the tongue tip (for production of the alveolar lateral /l/, Figure 5.6). Vocalic movements for the production of the vowel V1 were annotated on the movement trajectory of the tongue body.

For each articulatory movement three landmarks were defined in the vertical plane marking their position within the y-axis (cf. Section 3.2.3): i) start of movement (onset), ii) maximum target of movement, and iii) maximum speed (peak velocity). These landmarks were annotated by means of zero-crossings and maxima in the respective velocity trace (Figure 5.4).

Velocity problem

During the annotation process it became apparent that participants (speakers with PD and controls) sometimes produced deviant articulatory patterns when moving the tongue body towards its articulatory target. This was especially the case while producing vocalic sounds. The following scenarios occurred:

- Two or even more peaks in the velocity signal (Figure 5.5a).
- A velocity plateau (Figure 5.5b).

The phenomenon of multiple peaks is not new. As mentioned in section 3.3.1 and 4.1.4, multiple peaks in the velocity trace leading to submovements had been reported in older speakers (Mücke et al., 2021; Hermes et al., 2018) and speakers with dysarthria (Ziegler, 2002; Kent et al., 2000; Ackermann et al., 1995).

In the case of multiple peaks, one of them has to be selected for the analysis to guarantee consistency. For the purpose of this work the highest peak was chosen. If two peaks of the same height occurred, the first of the two was taken. When a velocity plateau was produced, its midpoint was chosen as the point of peak velocity. Regardless of which deviation occurs, it has an impact on the value of the peak velocity as well as on related measures.

Each decision on where to put the landmark has an impact on the duration of the acceleration and deceleration phase and on the movements' symmetry profile (ratio of deceleration/acceleration phase). Velocity profiles might therefore not be meaningful in these cases. But as peak velocity is an important parameter for describing a movement, the maximum speed will be reported. For the calculation of velocity profiles only bell-shaped velocity profiles of the vowels /i/ and /a/ are taken into account in the analysis.

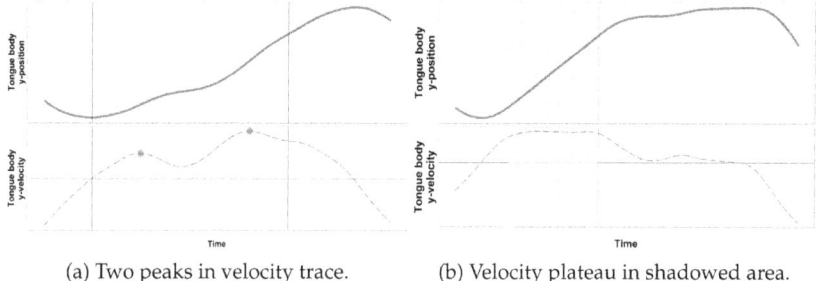

(a) Two peaks in velocity trace.   (b) Velocity plateau in shadowed area.

Figure 5.5. Examples of different velocity trajectories of a patient's tongue body movement. Vertical tongue position at the top and respective velocity trace below.

5.5.2 Measurements

As the main focus lies on the vocalic element within the first stressed syllable in this data set, most measurements were made by only considering measures related to vowel production. Moreover, as speech movements are reduced in the temporal and spatial dimension in speakers with PD, speech measures were applied to those dimensions of articulation (Duffy, 2019) as well as timing relations of underlying articulatory movements. The following acoustic and articulatory variables were computed:

Acoustic parameters

1. **Syllable duration** (ms): Temporal interval between the start of the first consonant C1 and the end of the first vowel V1 of the stressed syllable of each target word. Please note that this measure is only needed for the alignment measures discussed below and will not be reported alone.
2. **Acoustic vowel duration** (ms): Temporal interval between the start and the end of the first vowel V1 of each target word.

3. **Vowel Space Area:** The mean vowel formants F1 and F2 of the V1 vowels (/i, e, a, o, u/) were taken to represent the vowel space area. Vowel formants were calculated from the central 25 ms of the vocalic segment. Within this time frame, a formant value was taken every 6.25 ms respectively for F1 and F2. Finally, the average of all four values was calculated and taken as vowel formants F1 and F2 to plot the vowel space area (Boersma & Weenink, 2022).
4. **Vowel Articulation Index:** Based on the vowel formants F1 and F2 of the V1 vowels /i, a, u/, the Vowel Articulation Index (VAI) was calculated using the following formula (Sapir et al., 2010): $VAI = (F2_i + F1_a)/(F1_i + F1_u + F2_u + F2_a)$. This measure reflects vowel contrast and vowel centralization and has been shown to be sensitive to highly variable data and dysarthric speech. Higher values represent an enhancement of the vowel space.

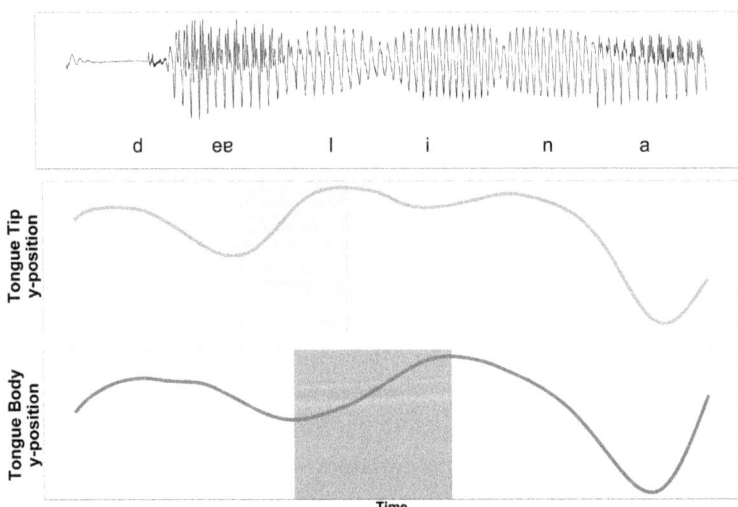

Figure 5.6. Acoustic waveform and movement trajectories of the tongue tip and the tongue body for the production of the utterance /deɐ linɐ/. The highlighted areas frame the interval from the onset to the maximum target per movement. The tongue tip (in light gray) is raised for /l/, and the tongue body (in dark gray) is raised for the vowel /i/.

Articulatory parameters

1. **Movement duration (ms):** Temporal interval between the onset of a movement and the maximum target (onset to target) indicating how much time the movement takes.
2. **Displacement (mm):** Relative positional difference between the onset and the maximum target of the movement on the vertical axis, indicating the spatial distance that has been traveled by the articulator.
3. **Peak velocity (mm/s):** Maximum speed of the movement between the onset and the target, indicating how fast a movement can be.
4. **Symmetry Profile:** The ratio of the deceleration phase to the acceleration phase. The temporal interval between the start of the movement to the maximum velocity (onset-to-peak velocity) corresponds to the acceleration phase of the movement, and the interval from the maximum velocity to the target of the movement (peak velocity to target) corresponds to the deceleration phase of the movement (cf. Section 3.2.3). Note that these parameters are only measured for tongue body movement producing the vowels /i/ and /a/.
5. **Stiffness:** Peak velocity divided by movement displacement (Munhall et al., 1985). The stiffer a movement is, the shorter it is, as it takes less time to achieve the articulatory target. This parameter will also be analyzed only for the vowels /i/ and /a/.

Whereas the articulatory parameters were computed for vocalic movements of the tongue body only, coordination measures also take into account the consonantal movement. To capture the timing relations of underlying movements, measures related to the initiation and coordination of movements were applied. As explained in chapter 3.2.4, the consonantal and the vocalic movement should start at the same time in a CV syllable, as they are timed in-phase (Browman & Goldstein, 1988). To additionally capture the coordination between underlying tongue kinematics and speech properties on the acoustic level, coordination patterns between landmarks of the vocalic movement and the acoustic syllable output are calculated, as it had been done in previous studies (cf. Thies et al., 2022, 2021). The expected coordination between articulatory movements and acoustic segments is depicted in Figure 5.7. The relevant measures are explained below:

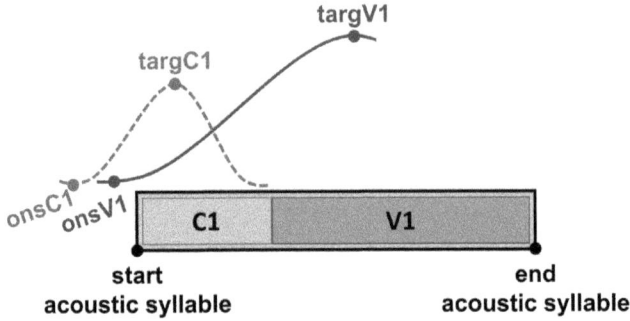

Figure 5.7. Coordination of articulatory movements and acoustic segments within a CV syllable.

Coordination parameters

1. **CV lag (ms):** Temporal interval between the onset of the consonantal movement (onsC1) and the onset of the vocalic movement (onsV1).
2. **TT lag (ms):** Temporal interval between the target of the consonantal movement (targC1) and the target of the vocalic movement (targV1).
3. **Onset Alignment:** Temporal interval between the onset of the vocalic tongue body movement (onsV1) and the left acoustic syllable boundary (start) divided by the acoustic syllable duration of the stressed CV syllable. Negative values indicate that the articulatory vocalic movement is initiated before the start of the acoustic syllable. The smaller the values, the earlier the movement is initiated before the start of the acoustic syllable.
4. **Target Alignment:** Temporal interval between the target of the vocalic tongue body movement (targV1) and the left acoustic syllable boundary (start) divided by the acoustic syllable duration of the stressed CV syllable. Positive values indicate an achievement within the acoustic syllable. The higher the values, the later the target is achieved within the acoustic syllable.

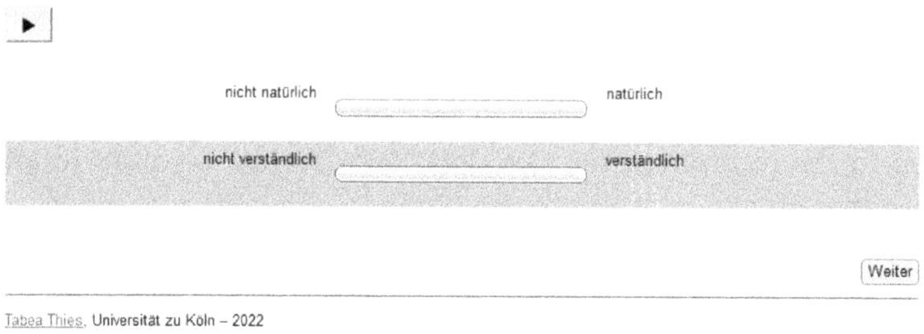

Speech Data Processing 111

Figure 5.8. Screenshot from SoSci Survey eliciting naive listener ratings. Clicking the play button started the audio.

Naive Listener Ratings

The collected speech data were presented to 165 naive listeners. They were asked to rate the naturalness and intelligibility of given speech samples produced by speakers with PD and healthy controls. The ratings were conducted with an online questionnaire using SoSci Survey (Leiner, 2019) that was distributed via Prolific (Prolific, 2014). The listeners were remunerated for their participation. Their task was to judge each speech sample on a scale from 1 to 101 with two two-sided VAS (Figure 5.8), ranging from not natural to natural, and from not intelligible to intelligible. Higher values indicate more natural and intelligible speech.

For the listener ratings, only productions in broad focus were selected as samples since they represented the most neutral condition. Moreover, only utterances containing target words with one of the three corner vowels /i, a, u/ as V1 of the stressed syllable were included. No added value is expected from including the inter-staged vowels /e/ and /u/. Moreover, this would significantly increase the scope of the perception experiment, which would have a negative impact on the informative value of the ratings, as listeners get exhausted and bored during the course of the experiment. The speech stimuli were divided into four experiments of equal size and were randomly presented to the 165 subjects. Therefore, each audio was rated at least 41 times. The participants were allowed to listen to the audio as many times as they wanted. Afterwards, they had to make a choice on both scales. Only when an answer was given it was possible to move on to the next audio. The subjects were encouraged to take a 5-minute break after the first and second third of the test. The total duration of the perception experiment was about 30 minutes.

Since the input level was adjusted for each participant and for each condition in the recordings, the raw data had different intensity levels. To ensure that all audios have a comparable level for the perceptual experiment, they were converged using the reference tones recorded as the first stimulus in each session. To scale the recordings to the same level, the intensity level of each reference tone was determined on the linear scale in Audacity (Audacity-Team, 2021). Then, the function "amplify" was used to set the new intensity level to 0.045 within the linear scale for all audios (Audacity-Team, 2021). The value for amplification was calculated using the formula: $20 * \log \frac{0.045}{reference}$.

The aim of this survey is to be able to assess changes in intelligibility and naturalness between speakers with PD and healthy controls, but also between the patients' therapeutic conditions.

5.6 Statistical Analysis

The data analysis was conducted using the statistical computing software R (version 4.1.2; R Core Team, 2022). Statistical analyses were performed for the following outcomes of interest: Motor functions, VAS ratings, acoustic measures (vowel duration, VAI), articulatory measures that describe movement patterns (duration, amplitude, velocity, symmetry, and stiffness), and measures related to articulatory timing (CV lag, TT lag, onset and target alignment).

In order to model motor functions (UPDRS III values) and to test differences between groups (CON vs PD) or treatment conditions (OFF vs ON) linear models were applied using the *lme4* package (Bates et al., 2015)[5]. Likelihood ratio tests were used to compare a null model that did not include the predictor (group or treatment) with an alternative model that did. Reported p-values are based on these comparisons.

The choice of a method for the analysis of visual analog scale (VAS) ratings is a controversial issue because there is no agreement on whether the outcome should be classified as ordinal or continuous

---

5   lm(UPDRS III score ~ group/treatment)

(Manuguerra et al., 2020). Taking this issue into account, a continuous ordinal regression model was used. This regression framework was applied to analyze speaker and listener ratings collected on a VAS by using the package *ordinalCont* (Manuguerra et al., 2020). For listener ratings, each rating category (intelligibility, naturalness) was taken as the outcome variable. Group or treatment condition were predictor variables. Random intercepts were included for speaker and rater[6]. To test the differences in the participants' self-perceived speaking ability, a fixed effect for group or treatment condition was included along with random intercepts for speakers. The coefficient estimates $\hat{\beta}$ and p-values that will be reported are taken from the model summaries.

In addition, a statistical analysis of acoustic and articulatory speech outcomes was performed with the *lme4* package (Bates et al., 2015). Linear mixed models were built with group (CON vs PD) or treatment condition (OFF vs ON) and focus type as predictor variables[7]. Random effects for varying intercepts and varying slopes were added per speaker conditioned on focus type (background, broad, contrastive) to account for speaker-specific prominence marking strategies. Random intercepts were included for vowel and consonant[8]. Please note that a reduced model was applied for testing the differences of the VAI, since only mean values per speaker and focus condition were available[9]. Interaction terms and main effects were validated by comparing the test model (with the interaction or critical predictor) to a reduced model (without the interaction or critical predictor) via likelihood-ratio tests. P-values are based on these comparisons. As none of the interaction terms of group/treatment x focus type were found significant, pairwise post-hoc analyses were completed by using the *emmeans* package (Lenth, 2022) if the main effects of the critical predictors were found significant.

---

6 ocm(intelligibility/naturalness ratings ~ group/treatment + (1|speaker) + (1|rater))
7 lmer(outcome ~ group/treatment * focus + (1+focus|speaker) + (1|vowel) + (1|consonant))
8 Target word was not included as a random effect because vowel and consonant already capture this.
9 lmer(VAI ~ group/treatment * focus + (1|speaker))

In addition, correlation coefficients are reported for some parameters. Normal distribution of the data was tested with the Shapiro-Wilk's test, and based on the results either a Pearson's or Spearman's correlation was applied. For each tested relationship, the type, coefficient and p-value are reported respectively. Given the small sample size and exploratory nature of the study, the alpha level of p < .05 was maintained and not corrected for multiple testing. Data files and R scripts are available in an open access GitHub repository via the following link: `https://github.com/TThies/dissertation-data`

6 Results: Disease Effect

As previously noted, this section will compare the speech of healthy control speakers and speakers with PD by investigating changes in the perceived intelligibility and naturalness as well as vowel production. To capture the disease effect, the speech of individuals with PD in medication-OFF condition (being off PD medication for at least 12 hours) is compared to that of healthy control speakers.

Articulatory speech patterns are analyzed in the temporal and spatial domain. With regard to the temporal domain, speakers with PD are expected to show slowed speech movements that are reflected in longer durational properties on the acoustic and articulatory level as well as reduced tongue body movement speeds. In parallel to the above mentioned slower articulation, a prolongation of deceleration phases, further indicating asymmetric movements, is also expected in speakers with PD.

In addition, movement amplitudes are expected to be smaller within an overall reduced and centralized articulation space. The reduction in the articulation space in speakers with PD should be reflected in a smaller vowel space and lower VAI values. If underlying articulatory movements are related to the acoustic and perceptual level, changes on the articulatory surface may influence the speech output that is perceived by listeners. As reduced movements are expected to result in less intelligible speech, it will be tested whether speech ratings correlate with articulatory features. Additionally, changes on the articulatory surface should influence the acoustic properties as well.

Moreover, it will be investigated whether articulatory impairment patterns are linked to specific motor symptoms. Especially, the relationship between pronounced axial deficits (or those who are related to posture and gait) and speech patterns will be investigated.

6.1 General Assessment

Data of 13 speakers with PD and 13 age- and sex-matched healthy controls were compared. Values yielded by the neuropsychological tests are given in the appendix A.2, as they were only used to exclude symptoms of depression and dementia. Cognitive values are not included in the following analysis.

Individuals with PD had been diagnosed with the disease 8 (SD = 5) years prior to being included in this study (Table 6.1). Their total UPDRS III score in medication-OFF condition ranged from 9 to 48, with an average of 25 (SD = 11). In contrast, values of the healthy controls ranged between 0 and 13, with a mean of 4 (SD = 4). UPDRS III values are about 21 points higher in the PD group compared to the control group. This difference is significant, as indicated by a linear model with group as predictor variable (F(-1) = 37.856, p < .001). When looking at UPDRS III subscores, individuals with PD do show axial impairment (axial: M = 4, SD = 3), problems with postural instability and gait (PIGD: M = 4, SD = 4) as well as higher bradykinesia scores (CON: M = 2, SD = 2 | PD: M = 10, SD = 7) and higher rigidity scores (CON: M = 2, SD = 2 | PD: M = 7, SD = 3) in comparison with control participants.

6.2 Speech Assessment

A speech therapist determined that all individuals with PD had mild dysarthric symptoms that were mainly related to speech tempo, articulation, voice quality, and prosody. Six patients talked with a slightly increased speech tempo and one with a reduced speech tempo accompanied by dysfluencies (PD11). Reduced articulatory precision and reduced prosodic modulations were reported for eight patients. Breathy and/or harsh voice was present in seven patients. Please note that the composition of dysarthric characteristics varies from speaker to speaker and that not every speaker had deficits in all domains. Table A.5 in the appendix gives an overview of the patients and their respective deficits. No swallowing difficulties have been reported by the patients themselves. Since speech problems were an exclusion criterion for the control speakers, no further information is provided on the speech characteristics for this group.

Speech Assessment 117

Table 6.1. Overview over general information of individuals with PD and age- and sex-matched healthy controls.

PD	sex	age	disease duration	UPDRS III	VAS	CON	sex	age	UPDRS III	VAS
PD01	m	69	13	48	7.4	CON01	m	69	22	7.3
PD02	f	51	6	23	8.4	CON02	f	48	2	7.7
PD03	m	63	10	15	6.5	CON03	m	62	5	7
PD04	m	54	5	22	7.4	CON04	m	55	2	7.3
PD05	m	68	12	39	7.5	CON05	m	67	11	6.7
PD06	m	56	5	16	10	CON06	m	57	6	8.6
PD07	f	70	20	11	10	CON07	f	71	11	6
PD08	m	53	4	29	6	CON08	m	53	2	8.8
PD09	f	69	13	27	5.5	CON09	f	67	9	3.6
PD10	m	42	7	34	7.1	CON10	m	45	1	6.2
PD11	m	59	4	23	9.5	CON11	m	58	2	10
PD12	m	56	7	14	3	CON12	m	57	12	8.4
PD13	f	56	2	9	9.5	CON13	f	59	-	7.8
mean (sd)	4 f, 9 m	59 (8)	8 (5)	25 (11)	7.3 (1.6)	*mean (sd)*	4 f, 9 m	59 (8)	4 (4)	7.4 (1.9)

6.2.1 Speech Ratings

Intelligibility and Naturalness

Less intelligible and less natural speech is expected in speakers with PD compared to healthy controls. The ratings of naive listeners verify this hypothesis, as not only intelligibility was rated lower in speakers with PD (CON: M = 85, SD = 18 | PD: M = 70, SD = 26) but also naturalness (CON: M = 78, SD = 22 | PD: M = 67, SD = 25). Intelligibility ratings are lowest in PD05 (M = 40, SD = 25) and highest in PD11 (M = 90, SD = 14). Naturalness ratings are lowest in PD11 (M = 36, SD = 28) and highest in PD03 (M = 78, SD = 18). The lowest rating for healthy controls is 71 in both categories.

Continuous ordinal regression models were applied to test whether listener ratings differ across the two groups. Each rating category was taken as the dependent variable, while group was taken as predictor variable. Random intercepts were included for speaker and rater. The models reveal lower intelligibility ($\hat{\beta} = 1.5$, $p < .001$) and less natural speech ($\hat{\beta} = 0.95$, $p < .001$) in speakers with PD.

VAS Ratings

The self-rated speaking ability, indicated by the VAS score, does not differ between both groups, with means and standard deviations being the same (Table 6.1). This is confirmed by a continuous ordinal regression model with group as predictor variable and speaker as random intercept ($\hat{\beta} = -0.13$, $p > .05$).

6.2.2 Acoustics

Vowel Duration

Individuals with dysarthria are expected to present slower articulation rates. Acoustic durations should therefore be longer in patients with PD compared to healthy controls. Likewise, longer acoustic durations are associated with an increase in prominence and should rise in both groups from background to broad and further to contrastive focus condition.

Figure 6.1 shows the acoustic durations of the vocalic segments within the stressed syllables for speakers with PD and healthy controls in each focus condition. The focus condition is color coded. Results of the control speakers are on the left, and results of the speakers with PD are on the right. A linear mixed model was applied to test if acoustic vowel durations differ between the two groups and whether the focus type has any influence. The main effects of group ($X^2(1) = 5.1666$, p = .023) and focus type ($X^2(2) = 31.407$, p < .001) were significant. Pairwise comparisons revealed that vowel durations are longer in speakers with PD compared to healthy control speakers (mean difference = 21 ms, p = .014). Moreover, prosodic adjustments were found in terms of increasing vowel durations from background to broad focus (mean difference = 12 ms, p < .001) and from background to contrastive focus (mean difference = 15 ms, p < .001). Vowel durations do not increase from broad to contrastive focus (mean difference = 3 ms, p > .05). This indicates that vowel durations are adjusted across but not within accentuation.

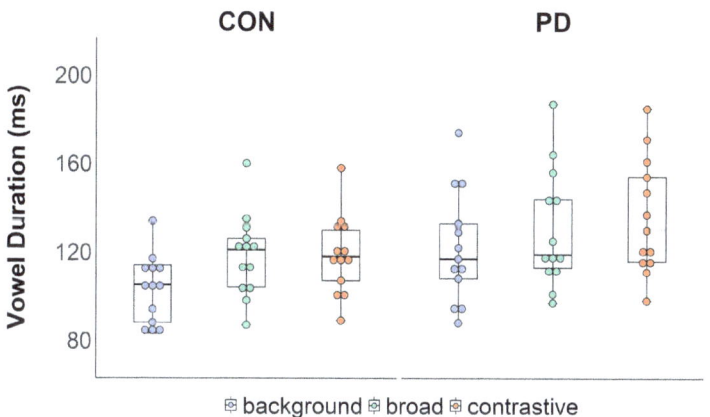

Figure 6.1. Acoustic vowel duration in ms per group and focus condition averaged across vowels and consonants.

Vowel Space

A reduced and centralized vowel space is expected in speakers with PD compared to healthy control speakers. In both groups the vowel space should increase under prominence due to hyper-articulation.

The Vowel Articulation Index (VAI) was calculated using the vowel formant frequencies F1 and F2 of the V1 vowels /i, a, o/. Higher values indicate larger vowel spaces. According to the values shown in Table 6.2, the vowel space appears to be smaller in speakers with PD. The reduction in vowel space can also be seen in Figure 6.2a. Here, the total vowel space area of both groups with all five corner vowels are compared across focus types. The vowel space area is smaller in the PD group (pink area) compared with the control group (gray area). While the linear mixed model comparison does not reveal a main effect of group ($X^2(1) = 1.4369$, $p > .05$), it does reveal a main effect of focus type ($X^2(2) = 10.758$, $p < .001$).

Table 6.2. Means and standard deviations of the Vowel Articulation Index for the control group and the PD group.

	Vowel Articulation Index	
	CON	PD
background	0.98 (0.08)	0.93 (0.12)
broad	1.01 (0.10)	0.97 (0.12)
contrastive	1.02 (0.09)	0.98 (0.14)
mean (sd)	1.00 (0.09)	0.96 (0.13)

With regard to prominence marking, pairwise post-hoc analyses reveal an increase of the VAI from background to broad focus (mean difference = 0.04, p = .032) and from background to contrastive focus (mean difference = 0.05, p = .005). However, the VAI does not increase from broad to contrastive focus (mean difference = 0.01, p > .05). This indicates that both groups only increase the vowel space across and not within accentuation. Further insights can be gathered from Figure 6.2b, which shows adjustment strategies per group. Focus types are color coded: background is blue, broad is green and contrastive is orange. The control speakers increase the vowel space to all sides equally under prominence. In the case of speakers with PD, the retraction of /u/ and /o/ is much stronger than the fronting of /i/ and /e/.

6.2.3 Articulation

Patterns of Tongue Body Movements

Tongue body movements during vowel production are analyzed with focus on movement duration, speed, and amplitude. Articulatory movements

Speech Assessment 121

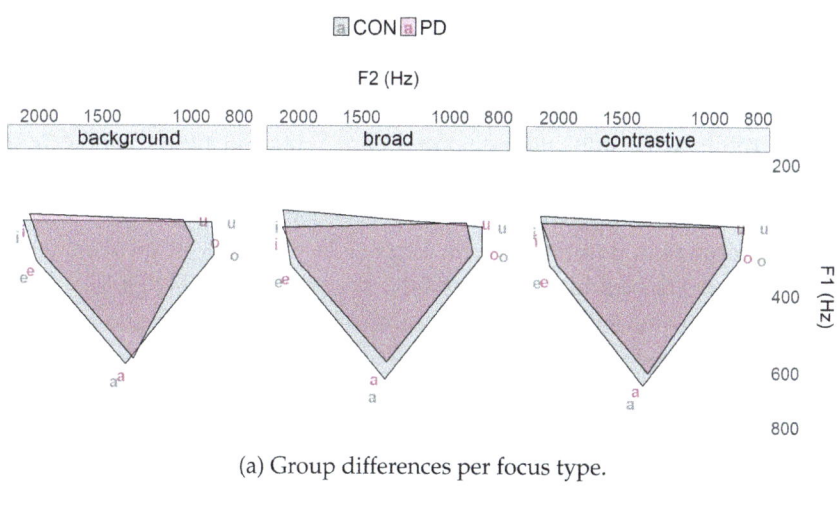

(a) Group differences per focus type.

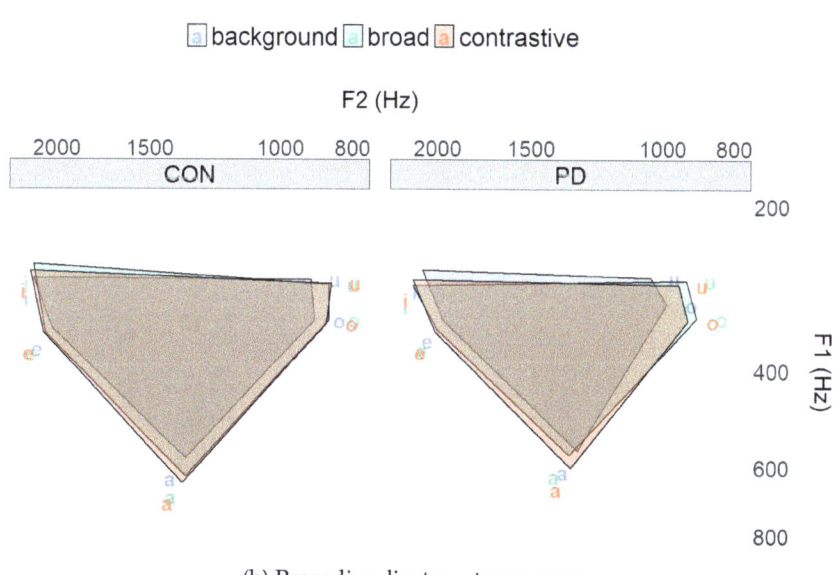

(b) Prosodic adjustments per group.

Figure 6.2. Vowel space area in healthy controls and speakers with PD.

are expected to be smaller in amplitude and to have slower velocities and longer durations.

Figure 6.3 presents averaged movement durations and movement amplitudes for each group and focus condition. Statistical analyses indicate a main effect of group ($X^2(1) = 5.8087$, $p < .016$) and focus type ($X^2(2) = 25.423$, $p < .001$) on movement durations. As can be seen from the figure, overall movement durations are on average 24 ms longer in speakers with PD compared to healthy controls (CON: M = 170, SD = 36| PD: M = 194, SD = 46). Movement durations are adjusted for prominence and increase from background to broad focus (mean difference = 11 ms, p = .003) and from background to contrastive focus (mean difference = 17 ms, p < .001).

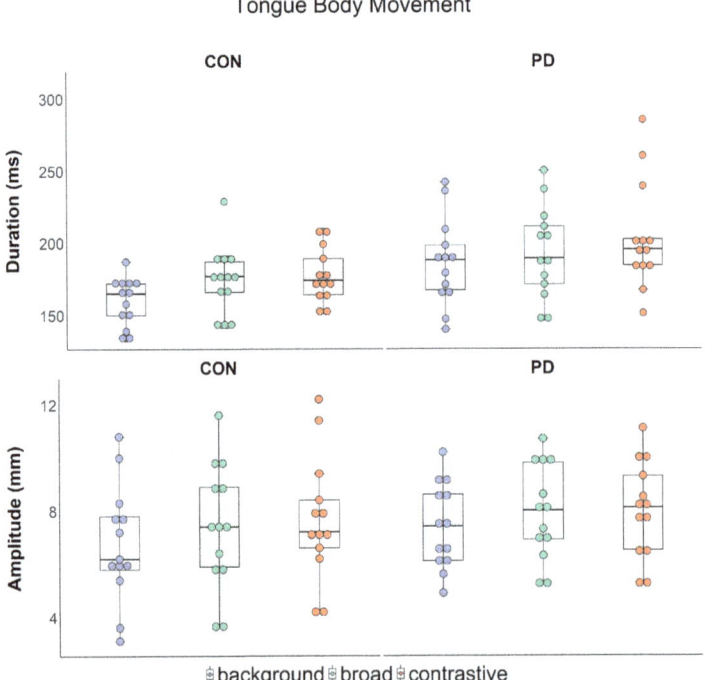

Figure 6.3. Tongue body movement duration and amplitude per focus condition comparing healthy control speakers and speakers with PD. Data is averaged across vowels and consonants.

On average, speakers with PD adjust movement durations from background to broad and further to contrastive focus condition (background: M = 186, SD = 43 | broad: M = 193, SD = 45 | contrastive: M = 203, SD = 49), whereas healthy controls only differentiate background and broad focus (background: M = 160, SD = 31 | broad: M = 174, SD = 40 | contrastive: M = 177, SD = 35). However, post-hoc comparisons do not indicate a change in movement duration from broad to contrastive focus (mean difference = 6 ms, p > .05). Thus, movement durations are adjusted across but not within accentuation.

Movement amplitudes are on average about 0.5 mm larger in the PD group compared to the control group (PD: M = 7.8, SD = 4.5 | CON: M = 7.3, SD = 4.2) but this difference is not significant ($X^2(1) = 0.6644$, p > .05). As it can be seen in the Figure 6.3, the distribution of data points is very variable, especially in the control group, as some speakers produced larger and others smaller amplitudes. However, there is a main effect of focus ($X^2(2) = 10.968$, p = .004). Pairwise comparisons reveal that amplitudes increase from background to broad focus (mean difference = 0.55 mm, p = .03) and from background to contrastive focus (mean difference = 0.71 mm, p = .004). Movement amplitudes do not change from broad to contrastive focus. Thus, movement amplitudes are adjusted across but not within accentuation.

Peak velocities do not differ between the groups (CON: M = 76, SD = 37 | PD: M = 74, SD = 41 | $X^2(1) = 0.0298$, p > .05) and are not adjusted under prominence ($X^2(2) = 1.9891$, p > .05). When comparing values for movement amplitude and velocity, some of the speakers presenting larger amplitudes also show faster velocities (PD05, CON11, PD12) and vice versa. Smaller and slower movements are seen in PD02, PD10, CON07 and CON13.

Another parameter of interest is the symmetry profile of tongue body movements, which is calculated as the ratio of deceleration phase to acceleration phase. Table 6.3 presents the respective values per group and focus condition. Only values for the production of the vowels /i/ and /a/ are considered. Overall phase durations are longer in the PD group, while the symmetry does not differ. The statistical analyses reveal no main effects for group ($X^2(1) = 0.0107$, p > .05) or focus type ($X^2(2) = 2.3559$, p > .05). In addition, the vowel productions' stiffness of /i/ and /a/ does neither differ across the groups (CON: M = 11.0, SD = 5 | PD: M = 9.3, SD = 2 | $X^2(1) = 2.2514$, p > .05) nor focus conditions (background: M = 9.7, SD = 1.9 | broad: M = 9.3, SD = 2.1 | contrastive: M = 9.0, SD = 2.1 | $X^2(2) = 2.713$, p > .05).

Table 6.3. Means and standard deviations for values describing the movement profile and corresponding phases in both groups. ACC = acceleration phase, DEC = deceleration phase, SYMM = symmetry profile.

	CON			PD		
	ACC	DEC	SYMM	ACC	DEC	SYMM
background	84 (29)	78 (21)	1.1 (0.6)	95 (34)	98 (33)	1.2 (0.6)
broad	92 (35)	96 (31)	1.2 (0.7)	102 (39)	102 (33)	1.2 (0.6)
contrastive	88 (31)	93 (31)	1.3 (0.8)	99 (31)	109 (39)	1.3 (0.7)
mean (sd)	88 (32)	89 (29)	1.2 (0.7)	99 (35)	103 (35)	1.2 (0.6)

Timing Relations of Tongue Body Movement

With respect to the acoustic syllable duration, the onset and target alignment of vocalic movements was calculated. Negative values indicate that the landmark lies before the start of acoustic syllable, positive values indicate an alignment within the syllable. Whereas the target alignment is expected to be stable, the onset initiation might vary in speakers with PD due to difficulties in initiating movements.

The target alignment is similar in both groups ($X^2(1) = 0.6523$, p > .05) and does not change with prosodic adjustments ($X^2(2) = 0.2312$, p > .05). The targets of vocalic tongue body movements are achieved at about 70 % (SD = 10) in the control group and at 69 % (SD = 11) in the PD group. This indicates similar target alignment patterns, although acoustic syllable durations are on average 28 ms longer in speakers with PD (CON: M = 196, SD = 37 | PD: M = 224, SD = 53). Not only the target achievement but also the initiation of movements seems to be timed consistently with respect to acoustic syllable duration, as there is neither a main effect of group ($X^2(1) = 0.3184$, p > .05) nor of focus condition ($X^2(2) = 4.3793$, p > .05). The vocalic target is initiated at -18 % (SD = 15) relative to the acoustic syllable start in healthy control speakers and at -19 % (SD = 17) in speakers with PD. In both groups, the consonantal movement is initiated before the vocalic movement and reaches its target earlier than the vocalic movement.

Whereas proportional timing patterns are stable and do not differ between the groups, the TT lag is larger in the PD group ($X^2(1) = 4.4016$, $p = .04$) because the consonantal and vocalic target lie further apart (CON: M = 104, SD = 32 | PD: M = 119, SD = 37). A significant difference of around 16 ms was estimated by the post-hoc comparison. In addition, the TT lag increases with prosodic adjustments ($X^2(2) = 21.873$, $p < .001$). While the TT lag increases from background to broad focus (mean difference = 10 ms, $p < .001$) and from background to contrastive focus (mean difference = 12 ms, $p < .001$), it does not differ between broad and contrastive focus (mean difference = 3 ms, $p > .05$), as pairwise comparisons reveal. In contrast, the main effects of group ($X^2(1) = 1.8463$, $p > .05$) and focus ($X^2(2) = 1.4016$, $p > .05$) were not found significant on the CV lag measure.

Correlations

The speech output (produced in broad focus) of speakers with PD is less intelligible compared with healthy control speakers. Therefore, the question arises which speech characteristics explain the reduced intelligibility.

Significant differences between the groups were found regarding acoustic vowel duration and tongue body movement duration. Longer vowel durations decrease intelligibility (Spearman: $r(75) = -.46$, $p < .001$) and also tend to decrease naturalness (Pearson: $r(75) = -.29$, $p = .011$) in healthy control speakers. In contrast, there is neither a correlation found between acoustic vowel durations and intelligibility ratings (Spearman: $r(74) = .10$, $p > .05$) nor between acoustic vowel durations and naturalness ratings (Spearman: $r(74) = -.23$, $p = .044$) in speakers with PD. Prolonged tongue movements decrease intelligibility in healthy control speakers (Spearman: $r(75) = -.30$, $p = .008$) but not in speakers with PD (Pearson: $r(75) = .06$, $p > .05$). This illustrates that any temporal prolongation reduces intelligibility in healthy speech. There is neither a relationship between tongue body movements and naturalness ratings in the control group

(Pearson: r(75) = -.12, p > .05) nor in the PD group (Spearman: r(74) = -.11, p > .05). In general, longer acoustic durations correlate with longer movement durations across all focus conditions in the control group (Spearman: r(232) = .57, p < .001) and in the PD group (Spearman: r(229) = .55, p < .001). Thus, articulatory changes in duration are reflected in the acoustic level.

VAI values tend to be smaller in speakers with PD indicating a reduced and centralized acoustic vowel space. Intelligibility scores in speakers with PD were found to be positively correlated with the VAI (Spearman: r(74) = .43, p < .001). This fits the initial hypothesis that a reduced articulation space decreases intelligibility. In addition, VAI values are positively correlated with naturalness ratings (Spearman: r(74) = .59, p < .001) in the PD group, pointing to the fact that as VAI values rise, speech is perceived as more natural. None of these correlation were found in the control group.

As motor functions are more impaired in the PD group, it will be investigated whether articulatory impairment patterns are linked to specific motor symptoms. Greater motor impairment leads to lower VAI values in the PD group. As various Spearman correlations reveal, this is true with regard to the total UPDRS III score (r(229) = -.39, p < .001) but also for the PIGD subscore (r(229) = -.54, p < .001), the axial subscore (r(229) = -.59, p < .001) and the bradykinesia subscore (r(229) = -.39, p < .001). This points to the fact that the size of the acoustic vowel space may serve as severity ratings of the disease. In contrast to spatial measurements, no temporal parameters are correlated with any of the motor symptoms.

6.3 Interim Conclusion

This chapter has shed light on the differences in acoustic, kinematic, and perceptual measures across prominence conditions between healthy control participants and individuals with PD. Based on the UPDRS III motor assessment, a greater motor impairment was determined for individuals with PD.

With regard to speech, the speech output of speakers with PD was rated as less intelligible and less natural compared with healthy control speakers. This decrease in intelligibility is based on a reduced acoustic vowel space and probably longer acoustic vowel durations in speakers with PD. In addition, greater motor impairments lead to a smaller acoustic vowel space.

Speakers with PD present longer tongue body movement durations that are also reflected in longer acoustic vowel durations. Proportional timing relations are apparently maintained regardless of the overall prolonged durations and do not differ between the two groups. Slowed movements increase the interval between the consonantal and the vocalic target in the PD group. Thus, overall longer durational properties are also reflected in the temporal intervals between articulatory landmarks. With regard to the spatial domain, no group differences were captured by the statistical analyses, but variation across speakers was identified. Trends can be observed towards larger tongue body movement amplitudes within an overall smaller acoustic vowel space.

With respect to prominence marking, both groups adjust speech parameters in the temporal and spatial domain. However, parameters are only adjusted across and not within accentuation in both speaker groups.

7 Results: Levodopa Effect

This part of the analysis is concerned with the potential effect of levodopa on speech parameters. Speakers with PD were recorded in two different conditions: without having taken any PD medication for at least 12 hours (med-OFF) and 30 to 40 minutes after having taken 200 mg of soluble levodopa (med-ON). As gross motor functions improve under levodopa, articulatory movements are expected to benefit from levodopa treatment as well.

It will be further investigated whether speech changes in underlying articulatory trajectories correspond to changes on the acoustic and perceptual level. Changes on the articulatory surface can be expected to influence acoustic properties, which should in turn impact how the speakers' output is perceived.

7.1 Motor Assessment

Individuals with PD were diagnosed 8 years (SD = 5) prior to study inclusion and had visible motor impairment. Figure 7.1 presents the scores of the UPDRS III motor assessment that was applied to capture changes in motor functions from med-OFF to med-ON condition. Each dot represents a patient per treatment condition. The treatment condition is color coded: med-OFF in pink and med-ON in green. Higher values indicate more severe motor impairment. UPDRS III scores in med-OFF condition range between 9 and 48, with an average of 25 (SD = 11). Under levodopa, the scores range between 6 and 19, with a mean of 11 (SD = 4). Thus, UPDRS III values are about 14 points lower in med-ON condition and drop in all individuals with PD from med-OFF to med-ON condition (Figure 7.1), with the only exception being PD13, whose values are the same across both conditions. She has a tremor-dominant PD type that is medication-refractory. The overall influence of levodopa on motor functions is supported by results from a linear model with treatment condition as predictor variable ($F(-1) = 17.855$, $p < .001$). The mean percentage of improvement is 49 % (SD = 24). All subscores responded similarly (axial: M = 49 %, SD = 44 | rigidity: M = 52 %, SD = 18 | bradykinesia: M = 54 %, SD = 30 | PIGD: M = 53 %, SD = 56).

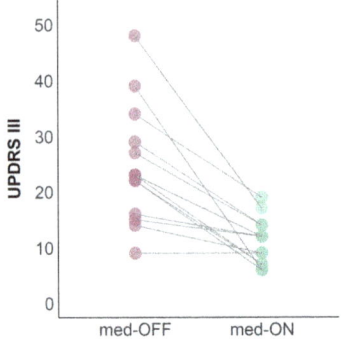

Figure 7.1. Visualization of the levodopa effect on motor functions per patient. Higher values indicate more pronounced motor impairment.

7.2 Speech Assessment

7.2.1 Speech Ratings

Intelligibility and Naturalness

Based on the previous literature reviewed, levodopa was not expected to lead to changes in perceived intelligibility or naturalness. However, intelligibility ratings are about 3 points higher in med-ON condition (med-OFF: M = 70, SD = 26 | med-ON: M = 73, SD = 24), while ratings of naturalness are identical in med-OFF and med-ON condition (med-OFF: M = 67, SD = 25 | med-ON: M = 67, SD = 25), according to the data analyzed.

This observation is confirmed by continuous ordinal regression models in which treatment condition (med-OFF vs med-ON) was included as predictor variable and speaker and rater as random intercepts. The models reveal higher intelligibility ($\hat{\beta}$ = -0.29, p < .001) in med-ON condition but unaltered naturalness ratings across treatment conditions ($\hat{\beta}$ = -0.03, p > .05).

VAS Ratings

The patients' self-rated speaking ability increased by 1.3 cm on the VAS in med-ON compared to med-OFF condition (med-OFF: M = 7.4, SD = 1.9 |

med-ON: M = 8.7, SD = 1.4). A continuous ordinal regression model with treatment condition as predictor variable and speaker as random intercept confirms this ($\hat{\beta}$ = -2.64, p = .003).

7.2.2 Acoustics

Vowel Duration

No effects on rate measures were observed in previous research. Therefore, no changes were expected in durational properties on the acoustic level due to levodopa intake.

Table 7.1 presents acoustic vowel durations in both treatment conditions averaged across all vowels and consonants. Vowel durations did not differ between med-OFF and med-ON condition as the main effect of treatment condition was not significant ($X^2(1) = 1.8629$, p > .05). However, the main effect of focus type was found significant ($X^2(2) = 20.403$, p < .001). Vowel duration increased by 10 ms from background to broad focus (p < .001), by 16 ms from background to contrastive focus (p < .001), and by 6 ms from broad to contrastive focus (p = .014), as pairwise comparisons revealed. This indicates that vowel durations are adjusted across and within accentuation.

Table 7.1. Means and standard deviations of acoustic vowel durations in ms per focus type in med-OFF and med-ON condition.

	Vowel Duration (ms)	
	med-OFF	med-ON
background	122 (33)	117 (32)
broad	130 (35)	130 (31)
contrastive	136 (36)	136 (33)
mean (sd)	129 (35)	128 (33)

Figure 7.2 depicts vowel durations in each focus condition and highlights the speaker-specific behavior. Each dot represents one speaker with PD per condition. As can be seen, one speaker with PD (PD11) presented overall longer vowel durations compared to all other speakers. On average, this speaker's vowel durations were 20 ms longer in med-OFF condition (M = 182, SD = 25) and 23 ms longer in med-ON condition

(M = 176, SD = 26) than those of the speaker with the second-longest vowel durations, whose values lie at the upper end of the remaining distribution (med-OFF: M = 162, SD = 37, med-ON: M = 153, SD = 29). The figure also indicates speaker-specific behavior in response to levodopa intake. Half of the patients increased vowel duration, while the other half decreased vowel duration respectively.

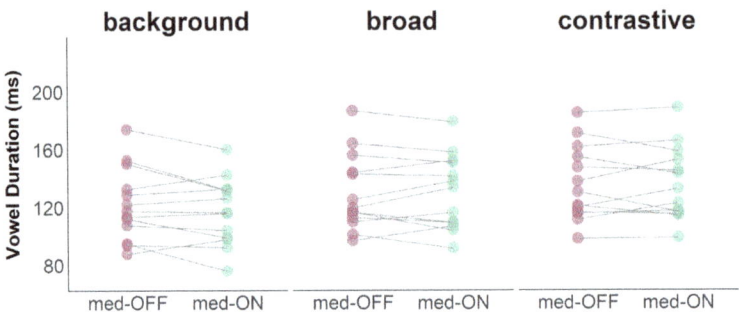

Figure 7.2. Acoustic vowel duration in ms per speaker with PD in each focus condition comparing med-OFF (pink) and med-ON (green) status.

Vowel Space

There is neither a main effect of treatment condition ($X^2(1) = 0.2405$, $p > .05$) nor of focus type on the VAI values ($X^2(2) = 3.9446$, $p > .05$). However, the data in med-ON condition is less variable, as the smaller standard deviations show (med-OFF: M = 0.96, SD = 0.13 | med-ON: M = 0.95 , SD = 0.08). The averaged VAI values indicate a tendency towards a smaller vowel space in prominent conditions in med-ON condition (background: M = 0.94, SD = 0.09 | broad: M = 0.95, SD = 0.08 | contrastive: M = 0.96, SD = 0.08) and less fine-grained prosodic modulations compared to med-OFF condition (background: M = 0.93, SD = 0.12 | broad: M = 0.97, SD = 0.12| contrastive: M = 0.98, SD = 0.14). The vowel space reduction in med-ON condition under prominence might be explained by a less strong retraction of the vowels /u/ and /o/, as can be seen in Figure 7.3. The figure presents the vowel space area outlined by vowel formants F1 and F2 of all five corner vowels in both treatment conditions separately. The three color-coded focus types show an increase in the vowel space area for prominent productions; from unaccented to accented productions in particular.

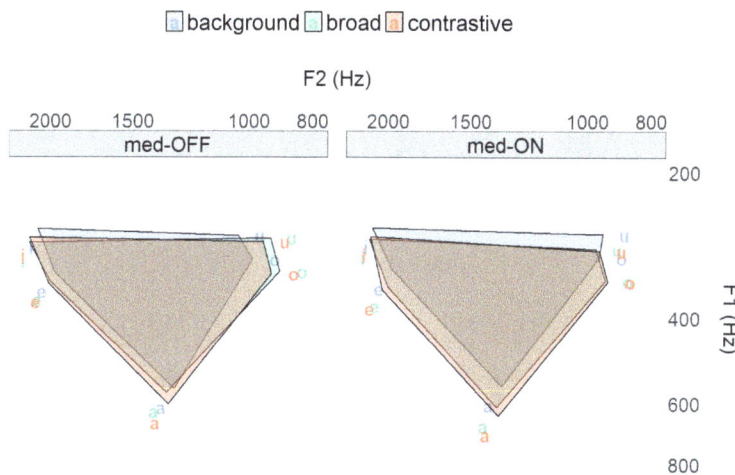

Figure 7.3. Prosodic adjustments within the vowel space area respectively per treatment condition: med-OFF on the left, med-ON on the right.

7.2.3 Articulation

Patterns of Tongue Body Movements

Based on the literature, faster and larger articulatory movements are expected under levodopa. Figure 7.4 depicts the results for tongue body movement measures in med-OFF and med-ON condition. Each color indicates one treatment condition. At first glance it looks like tongue body movements became shorter and faster in med-ON condition.

Statistical analyses reveal a main effect of treatment ($X^2(1) = 10.523$, $p = .001$) and focus type on movement duration ($X^2(2) = 10.408$, $p = .005$). Movement durations are on average 7 ms shorter under levodopa (med-OFF: M = 194, SD = 46 | med-ON: M = 187, SD = 47). In addition, pairwise comparisons reveal an increase in duration from background to broad focus (mean difference = 8 ms, p = .03) and from background to contrastive focus (mean difference = 15 ms, p = .005). No changes exist between broad and contrastive focus, indicating that movement durations are adjusted across but not within accentuation. With regard to movement amplitudes, there is no main effect of treatment (med-OFF: M = 7.8, SD = 4.5 | med-ON: M = 7.5, SD = 4.4 | $X^2(1) = 2.5105$, p > .05) but of focus type ($X^2(2) = 8.2281$, p = .02). However, movement amplitudes only increase from background to contrastive focus (mean difference = 0.6 mm, p = .007). The peak velocity does neither change under levodopa (med-OFF: M = 74, SD = 41 | med-ON: M = 77, SD = 44 | $X^2(1) = 3.4058$, p > .05), nor under prominence ($X^2(2) = 2.3969$, p > .05).

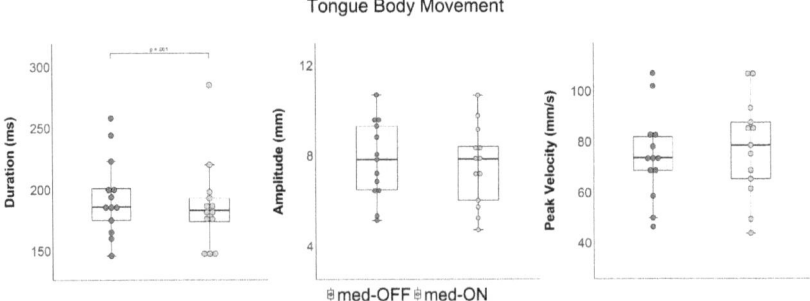

Figure 7.4. Tongue body movement patterns in med-OFF and med-ON condition averaged across focus types, vowels, and consonants.

However, patients responded differently to levodopa intake, as seven speakers decreased movement durations in med-ON condition, whereas six increased movement durations. Two extreme examples are PD11, who increased movement durations by 27 ms on average, and PD09 who shortened durations by -35 ms. The same heterogeneity was found for movement amplitude and velocity. Whereas seven speakers produced larger amplitudes and five smaller amplitudes under levodopa, eight speakers produced faster and five slower tongue body movements under levodopa. Please note that not all speakers who showed larger amplitudes after taking levodopa also produced faster movements. When all three parameters are analyzed together, different patterns of change become visible. Six patients showed longer, larger, and faster tongue body movements in med-ON condition (e.g., PD05, PD06, PD07, PD08). In contrast, three patients produced shorter, smaller, and slower movements (PD01, PD02, PD04). Whereas in PD10 and PD11 parameters are only changed in the temporal domain (shorter and slower), two other speakers (PD03, PD09) make adjustments in the temporal and the spatial domain, producing longer, smaller, and faster movements under levodopa.

The shortening in the temporal domain is also reflected in shorter acceleration phases in med-ON condition, which were about 7 ms shorter during the production of the vowels /i/ and /a/ (Table 7.2). With regard to prominence marking, movement durations increased across accentuation. This prolongation can also be found in deceleration phases, especially in med-ON condition (Table 7.2). However, the overall symmetry profile remained unchanged regardless of treatment condition ($X^2(1) = 0.3965$, $p > .05$) and focus type ($X^2(2) = 2.1199$, $p > .05$).

Table 7.2. Means and standard deviations for values describing the movement profile and corresponding phases in med-OFF and med-ON condition. ACC = acceleration phase, DEC = deceleration phase, SYMM = symmetry profile.

	med-OFF			med-ON		
	ACC	DEC	SYMM	ACC	DEC	SYMM
background	95 (34)	98 (33)	1.2 (0.6)	91 (31)	93 (28)	1.2 (0.5)
broad	102 (39)	102 (33)	1.2 (0.6)	94 (35)	100 (35)	1.2 (0.7)
contrastive	99 (31)	109 (39)	1.3 (0.7)	91 (30)	108 (42)	1.3 (0.7)
mean (sd)	99 (35)	103 (35)	1.2 (0.6)	92 (32)	100 (36)	1.2 (0.6)

Stiffness was lower in med-OFF condition during the production of the vowels /i/ and /a/ (med-OFF: M = 9.3, SD = 2.0 | med-ON: M = 9.8, SD = 2.1 | $X^2(1) = 4.7657$, p = .03), indicating a significant change in speech effort under levodopa. However, stiffness was not used to encode prominence ($X^2(1) = 4.1496$, p > .05).

Timing Relations of Tongue Body Movement

Onset and target alignment was calculated in proportion to the acoustic syllable duration. Negative values indicate that the respective landmark lies before the start of the acoustic syllable, positive values indicate an alignment within the syllable. Whereas a stable target alignment was expected across treatment conditions, the initiation of movements might be later in med-ON condition due to improved speech planning abilities.

The target alignment was stable across the two treatment conditions. Vocalic targets were achieved within 68.5 % (med-OFF: M = 69, SD = 11 | med-ON: M = 68, SD = 11) of the total syllable duration. There was neither a main effect of treatment ($X^2(1) = 0.9405$, p > .05) nor of focus ($X^2(2) = 0.0384$, p > .05) found on the target alignment measure. In contrast, the onset was timed later with respect to the syllable in med-ON condition (med-OFF: M = -19 %, SD = 17 | med-ON: M = -17 %, SD = 14 | $X^2(1) = 5.9861$, p = .014). In addition, tongue body movement initiation differed with regard to prosodic adjustments ($X^2(2) = 9.5144$, p = .009). Post-hoc comparisons reveal a change from background to contrastive focus, with later initiation in the prominent condition (mean difference = 3 %, p = .006). Onset initiation did neither differ across background and broad focus nor within accentuation.

While the CV lag does neither differ between med-OFF and med-ON condition ($X^2(1) = 0.0411$, p > .05) nor between focus types ($X^2(2) = 2.2874$, p > .05), the TT lag changes under levodopa ($X^2(1) = 4.198$, p = .041) and under prominence ($X^2(2) = 14.67$, p < .001). Vocalic movements were on average initiated 27.5 ms after consonantal movements (med-OFF: M = 27, SD = 36 | med-ON: M = 28, SD = 34) and vocalic targets were achieved 117 ms after consonantal targets (med-OFF: M = 119, SD = 37 | med-ON: M = 115, SD = 38). The shortening on the temporal level is also reflected in the TT lag, as this is 4 ms shorter under levodopa. Under prominence, the TT lag increased from background to broad focus (mean difference = 8 ms, p = .008) and from background to contrastive focus (mean difference = 14 ms, p < .001). The TT lag does not change within accentuation.

7.3 Correlations

The speech output of speakers with PD was found to be more intelligible after levodopa intake. In the following, speech characteristics explaining the improved intelligibility in med-ON condition will be explored.

The result of the previous chapter propose that a larger acoustic vowel space and shorter vowel durations should lead to higher intelligibility ratings.

However, none of the speech parameters were shown to correlate with intelligibility in med-ON condition. Regarding naturalness, results suggest that acoustic vowel durations (Spearman: $r(74) = -.42$, $p < .001$) and tongue body movement durations (Spearman: $r(74) = -.38$, $p < .001$) are negatively correlated with naturalness ratings. Thus, prolonged durational properties decrease the perceived naturalness. In addition, longer acoustic durations correlate with longer movement durations across all focus conditions (Spearman: $r(228) = .60$, $p < .001$). In addition, there is a trend that VAI values are correlated with naturalness (Spearman: $r(74) = .25$, $p = .027$), indicating that a smaller vowel space decreases naturalness.

No clear relationships between speech parameters and motor scores could be detected in med-ON condition. However, as the patients' self-rated VAS scores was higher in med-ON condition, it will be investigated which parameters correlate with the VAS score. Spearman correlations revealed a trend towards a positive relationship between VAS ratings and acoustic vowel durations ($r(228) = .28$, $p < .001$) and towards a negative relationship between VAS ratings and axial motor symptoms ($r(74) = .28$, $p = .013$). Thus, longer acoustic vowel durations and less axial impairment lead to the higher VAS ratings.

7.4 Interim Conclusion

Motor functions improved under levodopa and naive listeners rated the speech output as more intelligible. This change in speech production was also recognized by the speakers themselves, as their ratings of their own speaking ability improved.

While the target alignment does not change under levodopa, the initiation of vocalic tongue body movements occurred later in med-ON condition possibly due to improved speech planning abilities. While shorter tongue body durations were found on the articulatory level, this change was not reflected in acoustic vowel durations. Moreover, no significant changes could be detected from med-OFF to med-ON condition with regard to movement amplitude or peak velocity. However, trends towards shorter, smaller, and faster movements are visible, which consequently increase the movements' stiffness. When investigating individual responses, the majority of patients actually show longer, larger, and faster movements under levodopa, and thereby enhance the entire articulatory movement respectively.

Under prominence, durational properties increased across and within accentuation on the acoustic level but only across accentuation on the articulatory level. A different pattern can be determined for spatial modulations, as the VAI was not at all adjusted under prominence, while the movement amplitude increased across accentuation.

8 Results: DBS Effect

To capture the treatment effect of STN-DBS, speakers with PD were recorded in two conditions: with deactivated stimulation (DBS-OFF) and with activated stimulation (DBS-ON). In both conditions, patients had not taken any PD drugs for 12 hours prior to participating in the study. Since one participant did not tolerate the DBS-OFF condition, only twelve individuals with PD are included in this analysis.

As gross motor functions are improved under DBS treatment, articulatory movements are expected to benefit as well although the effect is inconclusive in the literature. As before, it will be investigated whether speech changes in underlying articulatory trajectories correspond to changes on the acoustic and perceptual level. Changes on the articulatory surface can be expected to influence acoustic properties, which should in turn impact how the speakers' output is perceived.

8.1 Motor Assessment

Post-surgery assessments were done on average 9 months (SD = 3) after the implantation of STN-DBS. Figure 8.1 presents the scores of the UPDRS III motor assessment, which was applied to capture changes in motor functions from DBS-OFF to DBS-ON condition per patient. Each dot represents one patient, and the treatment condition is color coded: DBS-OFF in blue and DBS-ON in brown. Higher values are related to greater motor impairment. The total UPDRS III scores in DBS-OFF condition range between 15 and 40 with an average of 26 (SD = 9). With activated stimulation, the scores range between 3 and 34 with a mean of 13 (SD = 9). Thus, UPDRS III values are about 13 points lower in DBS-ON condition. This is confirmed by the linear model ($F_{(-1)} = 13.22$, $p < .001$) with treatment condition as predictor variable. With the exception of one participant (PD07 changes only from 19 to 18 points), all patients have lower UPDRS III scores in DBS-ON condition (Figure 8.1). The mean improvement is about 50 % (SD = 25). However, subscores behave differently, with rigidity showing the greatest response (M = 66 %, SD = 21), followed by bradykinesia (M = 47 %, SD = 29) and axial symptoms (M = 31 %, SD = 51). PIGD scores do not change on average.

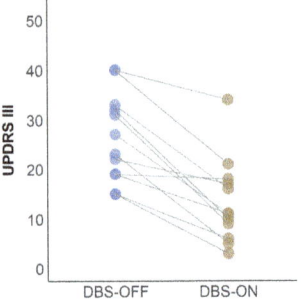

Figure 8.1. Visualization of the DBS effect on motor functions per patient. Higher values indicate more pronounced motor impairment.

8.2 Speech Assessment

8.2.1 Speech Ratings

Intelligibility and Naturalness

Intelligibility ratings are higher with activated DBS compared to deactivated DBS (DBS-OFF: M = 69, SD = 26 | DBS-ON: M = 71, SD = 26), as confirmed by a continuous ordinal regression model ($\hat{\beta}$ = -0.24, p < .001). In contrast, naturalness ratings do not differ between DBS-OFF and DBS-ON condition (DBS-OFF: M = 67, SD = 26 | DBS-ON: M = 65, SD = 28 | $\hat{\beta}$ = 0.07, p > .05). In both continuous ordinal regression models each rating category was taken as the dependent variable and treatment condition (DBS-OFF vs DBS-ON) as predictor variable. Random intercepts were included for speaker and rater.

VAS Ratings

The VAS score is higher in DBS-ON condition than in DBS-OFF condition (DBS-OFF: M = 5.8, SD = 3.0 | DBS-ON: M = 7.4, SD = 2.2). This indicates that the speakers themselves perceived their speaking ability to be better with activated DBS. A continuous ordinal regression model with treatment condition as predictor variable and speaker as random intercept supports this observation ($\hat{\beta}$ = -1.94, p = .018).

8.2.2 Acoustics

Vowel Duration

Vowel durations are reported in Table 8.1 per treatment condition and focus type averaged across vowels and consonants. While the main effect of treatment condition was not significant ($X^2(1)$ = 0.8774, p > .05), the main effect of focus type was significant ($X^2(2)$ = 30.904, p < .001). Thus, vowel durations do not change from DBS-OFF to DBS-ON condition but are adjusted under prominence. Pairwise post-hoc analyses reveal that vowel durations increase from background to broad focus (mean difference = 13 ms, p < .001), from background to contrastive focus (mean difference = 20 ms, p < .001), and from broad to contrastive focus (mean difference = 6 ms, p = .005). This indicates that vowel durations are adjusted across and within accentuation. Moreover, durational adjustments across accentuation are greater after surgery than before it.

Table 8.1. Means and standard deviations of acoustic vowel durations in ms per focus condition in DBS-OFF and DBS-ON.

	Vowel Duration (ms)	
	DBS-OFF	DBS-ON
background	129 (33)	127 (38)
broad	141 (38)	141 (42)
contrastive	149 (39)	146 (37)
mean (sd)	140 (37)	138 (40)

Figure 8.2 depicts vowel durations in each focus condition and highlights the speaker-specific behavior related to treatment condition. Similarly to what was found in the preoperative assessment, half of the patients increase vowel duration under activated DBS, the other half decreases vowel duration respectively. In addition, speaker PD11 produced overall longer vowel durations compared to all other speakers. On average, this patient's vowel durations are 21 ms longer in DBS-OFF condition (M = 186, SD = 31) and 48 ms longer in DBS-ON condition (M = 212,

SD = 19) than those of the speaker who presented the next-highest value (DBS-OFF: M = 165, SD = 32 | DBS-ON: M = 164, SD = 27). The speaker stands out from the group even more than in the preoperative measurements.

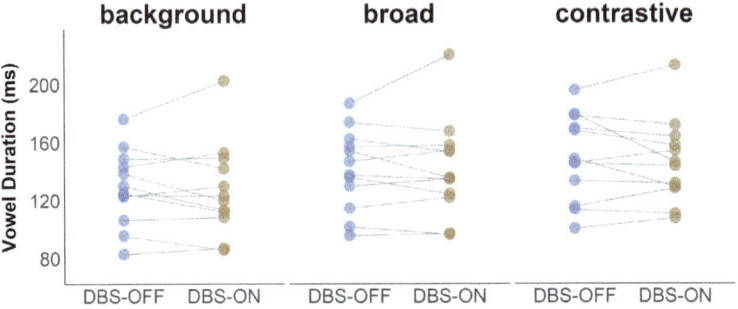

Figure 8.2. Acoustic vowel duration in ms per speaker with PD in each focus condition. Respectively with deactivated (DBS-OFF, blue) and activated stimulation (DBS-ON, brown).

Vowel Space

The VAI does not differ between the two treatment conditions (DBS-OFF: M = 0.95, SD = 0.09 | DBS-ON: M = 0.94, SD = 0.09 | $X^2(1) = 0.4425$, p > .05). It seems that the VAI values increase across accentuation in both DBS-OFF condition (background: M = 0.93, SD = 0.11 | broad: M = 0.95, SD = 0.09 | contrastive: M = 0.96, SD = 0.09) and DBS-ON condition (background: M = 0.92, SD = 0.08 | broad: M = 0.94, SD = 0.09 | contrastive: M = 0.94, SD = 0.10). However, the linear mixed model comparison does not reveal a main effect for prosodic adjustments ($X^2(2) = 1.9426$, p > .05).

8.2.3 Articulation

Patterns of Tongue Body Movements

Shorter and larger tongue movements can be expected under activated DBS. However, the data shows that tongue body movements do not change with activated DBS. Movement durations are the same in DBS-OFF and DBS-ON condition (DBS-OFF: M = 194, SD = 46 | DBS-ON: M = 198, SD = 55), as confirmed by the linear mixed model comparison ($X^2(1) = 0.868$, p > .05). However, there is a main effect of focus type ($X^2(2) = 17.706$, p < .001). Pairwise post-hoc comparisons indicate an increase in movement duration from background to broad focus (mean difference: 10 ms, p = .009) and from background to contrastive focus (mean difference = 16 ms, p < .001). Movement durations do not change from broad to contrastive focus. Thus, movement durations are adjusted across but not within accentuation. Prosodic changes are comparable with those at the preoperative visit.

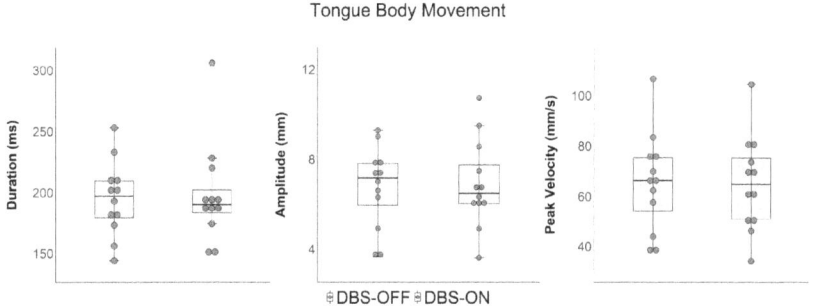

Figure 8.3. Tongue body movement patterns in DBS-OFF and DBS-ON condition averaged across focus types, vowels, and consonants.

Neither the amplitude of tongue body movements (DBS-OFF: M = 6.8, SD = 4.4 | DBS-ON: M = 6.9, SD = 4.6 | $X^2(1) = 0.053$, p > .05) nor the average peak velocities changed under activated DBS (DBS-OFF: M = 66, SD = 40 | DBS-ON: M = 65, SD = 39 | $X^2(1) = 0.3772$, p > .05), according to the model comparisons. Moreover, both parameters were not adjusted under prominence (amplitude: $X^2(2) = 5.6$, p > .05 | peak velocity: $X^2(2) = 0.7261$, p > .05).

An inspection of individual responses reveals heterogeneous patterns across patients. It becomes visible that eight speakers shorten durations and only four speakers prolong durations in DBS-ON condition. The prolongation is particularly pronounced in PD11. Most of the patients that show shorter durations also produce smaller movements (PD01, PD04, PD05, PD07, PD08, PD09). Longer movements go along with larger movements in speakers PD02, PD10, PD11, and PD13. Two speakers have shorter but larger movements in DBS-ON condition (PD06, PD12).

The prolongation under prominence in the temporal domain can also be determined for underlying movement phases in the vowels /i/ and /a/. Especially a prolongation of the deceleration phases led to more asymmetrical movements under prominence (Table 8.2). However, the overall symmetry profile remained unchanged regardless of treatment condition ($X^2(1) = 0.0257$, $p > .05$) and focus type ($X^2(2) = 1.8279$, $p > .05$). In addition, the movements' stiffness remains the same in productions of the vowels /i/ and /a/ (DBS-OFF: M = 9.6, SD = 2.5 | DBS-ON: M = 9.8, SD = 2.7 | $X^2(1) = 1.3287$, $p > .05$) and does not change under prominence ($X^2(2) = 3.3107$, $p > .05$).

Table 8.2. Means and standard deviations for values describing the movement profile and corresponding phases comparing DBS-OFF and DBS-ON condition. ACC = acceleration phase, DEC = deceleration phase, SYMM = symmetry profile.

	DBS-OFF			DBS-ON		
	ACC	DEC	SYMM	ACC	DEC	SYMM
background	95 (40)	97 (25)	1.2 (0.6)	98 (37)	99 (31)	1.2 (0.7)
broad	100 (39)	107 (29)	1.3 (0.7)	100 (44)	107 (39)	1.3 (0.8)
contrastive	97 (37)	111 (30)	1.3 (0.7)	102 (42)	110 (42)	1.3 (0.7)
mean (sd)	97 (39)	105 (29)	1.3 (0.7)	100 (41)	105 (38)	1.2 (0.7)

Timing Relations of Tongue Body Movement

Onset and target alignment was calculated in proportion to the acoustic syllable duration. Negative values indicate that the respective landmark lies before the start of the acoustic syllable, positive values indicate an alignment within the syllable.

One interesting observation was that the timing patterns of patients in DBS-ON condition were comparable to the alignment patterns of healthy controls. Especially the onset alignment was similar, with vocalic movements being initiated 18 % before the start of the acoustic syllable in both groups. The CV lag between consonantal and vocalic onsets was also comparable in both groups (CON: M = 20 ms, SD = 32 | DBS-ON: M = 24 ms, SD = 34).

Neither the alignment of vocalic onsets (DBS-OFF: M = -16, SD = 15 | DBS-ON: M = -18, SD = 14 | $X^2(1) = 3.057$, p > .05) nor of vocalic targets (DBS-OFF: M = 68, SD = 10 | DBS-ON: M = 68, SD = 9 | $X^2(1) = 1.212$, p > .05) change from DBS-OFF to DBS-ON in speakers with PD and seem stable across treatment conditions. In addition, both alignment patterns are not adjusted under prominence (onset: $X^2(2) = 4.9699$, p > .05 | target: $X^2(2) = 0.2492$, p > .05).

However, the time interval between landmarks of the vocalic and the preceding consonantal movement changes in DBS-ON condition. The CV lag was smaller, indicating that the initiation of the consonantal and the vocalic movement were closer to one another when DBS was activated (DBS-OFF: M = 31, SD = 38 | DBS-ON: M = 24, SD = 34 | $X^2(1) = 8.836$, p = .003). Prosodic adjustment did not lead to any changes ($X^2(2) = 1.2334$, p > .05). The time interval between both targets (TT lag) decreased by 5 ms under activated DBS (DBS-OFF: M = 125, SD = 34 | DBS-ON: M = 121, SD = 36 | $X^2(1) = 5.7872$, p = .016). Prosodic adjustments, on the other hand, lead to an increase of the TT lag ($X^2(2) = 19.811$, p > .05) across and within accentuation. The TT lag increases by 8 ms from background to broad focus (p = .005), by 15 ms from background to contrastive focus (p < .001), and by 7 ms from broad to contrastive focus (p = .014).

8.3 Correlations

The speech output of speakers with PD was more intelligible in DBS-ON condition than in DBS-OFF condition. This raises the question of which speech characteristics explain the improved intelligibility under activated DBS.

The results of a Spearman correlation revealed that there was a positive correlation between intelligibility ratings and VAI values (r(75) = .50, p < .001). Thus an increase in vowel space increases perceived intelligibility. However, none of the other parameters were shown to correlate with intelligibility. On the contrary, an increase in naturalness can be achieved by shortening acoustic vowel durations and by increasing the vowel space, as acoustic vowel duration was negatively (r(75) = -.40, p < .001) and VAI values positively (r(75) = .47, p < .001) correlated with naturalness ratings, as Spearman correlations indicated. Again, longer acoustic durations correlate with longer movement durations across all focus conditions (Spearman: r(214) = .62, p < .001).

VAI values were higher when axial motor symptoms (Spearman: r(214) = -.30, p < .001) and PIGD motor symptoms are less pronounced (r(214) = -.32, p < .001). This points to the fact that the size of the acoustic vowel space may serve as severity ratings of the disease. No clear relationships between other speech parameters and motor scores could be detected in DBS-ON condition. As the patients' self-rated VAS scores was higher in med-ON condition, it will be investigated which parameters correlate with the VAS score. Lower motor impairment led to the higher VAS ratings, as indicated by Spearman correlations for the total UPDRS III scores (r(76) = -.58, p < .001) and the axial subscores (r(76) = -.43, p < .001). Moreover, VAS scores increase with longer durations (TB duration: r(232) = .32, p < .001 | V1 duration: r(232) = .34, p < .001) and higher VAI values (r(232) = .37, p < .001).

8.4 Interim Conclusion

Activated DBS improved motor functions and increased the perceived intelligibility. Changes were perceived by the patients themselves, as they gave their speaking ability better ratings in DBS-ON condition.

No significant changes from DBS-OFF to DBS-ON condition could be detected regarding speech parameters. But there was a noticeable trend towards shorter and smaller movements under DBS for the majority of patients. The shortening was also reflected in the time interval between the articulatory landmarks of the vowel and the preceding consonant, as not only the initiation but also the reaching of the target of both movements were closer together when DBS was activated.

Only acoustic vowel durations and tongue body movement durations were adjusted under prominence, while spatial parameters were not modulated.

9 Results: Levodopa vs STN-DBS

This chapter is concerned with the question of whether one treatment is superior to the other. The aim is to determine whether parameters of interest change to the same extent following levodopa intake and STN-DBS. To this end, a comparison between the two ON conditions, med-ON and DBS-ON, will be made. The preoperative med-OFF condition will be considered as the baseline.

9.1 Motor Assessment

As it was shown earlier, both levodopa and STN-DBS improve motor functions. Percentagewise, the improvement from med-OFF to med-ON is 49 % (SD = 24). Subscores of the UPDRS III show the same or higher improvement under levodopa (axial: M = 49 %, SD = 44 | rigidity: M = 52 %, SD = 18 | bradykinesia: M = 54 %, SD = 30 | PIGD: M = 53 %, SD = 56). When comparing the total raw score of 25 (SD = 11) in med-OFF to 14 (SD = 9) in DBS-ON, the percentage change is 38 % (SD = 39). Therefore, the DBS effect is smaller than the levodopa effect when compared to the preoperative baseline condition. Moreover, most of the subscores do not change from baseline to DBS-ON. Only rigidity seems to improve by 56 % (SD = 52) from med-OFF to DBS-ON.

9.2 Speech Assessment

9.2.1 Speech Ratings

Intelligibility and Naturalness

As presented in chapter 7, intelligibility increases from med-OFF to med-ON condition ($\hat{\beta}$ = -0.29, p < .001). When comparing med-OFF to DBS-ON, intelligibility also increases ($\hat{\beta}$ = 0.17, p < .001). Thus, intelligibility improves with treatment, but the difference that levodopa causes is greater (+3) than that of DBS (+1). In contrast, naturalness neither changes from med-OFF to med-ON ($\hat{\beta}$ = -0.03, p > .05) nor from med-OFF to DBS-ON ($\hat{\beta}$ = -0.07, p > .05), according to the listeners' ratings.

VAS Rating

The patients' self-rated VAS scores are lowest in med-OFF condition (M = 7.4, SD = 1.9). Following both treatments, only levodopa resulted in higher VAS ratings compared to med-OFF condition (med-ON: M = 8.7, SD = 1.4 | DBS-ON: M = 7.5, SD = 2.2). In line with this observation, only the difference in VAS score induced by levodopa intake is significant, according to results from a continuous ordinal regression model with treatment condition as predictor variable and speaker as random intercept (med-OFF vs med-ON: $\hat{\beta}$ = -2.64, p = .003 | med-OFF vs DBS-ON: $\hat{\beta}$ = -0.32, p > .05).

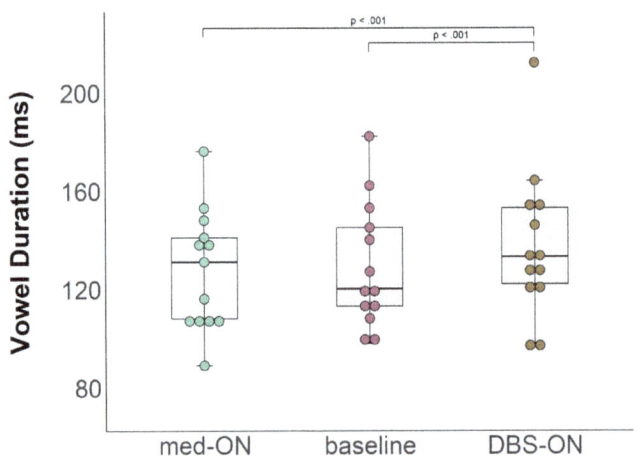

Figure 9.1. Changes in acoustic vowel duration in relation to both treatments compared to the preoperative baseline (med-OFF). Levodopa effect: baseline to med-ON condition. DBS-effect: baseline to DBS-ON condition.

9.2.2 Acoustics

Vowel Duration

Figure 9.1 compares the acoustic vowel duration from baseline to med-ON condition and from baseline to DBS-ON condition averaged across focus types, vowels, and consonants. The preoperative med-OFF condition is taken as the baseline. Therefore, changes from baseline to med-ON, on the left side, show the levodopa effect, while changes from baseline to DBS-ON, on the right side, highlight the DBS effect.

There is a main effect of treatment on acoustic vowel durations ($X^2(2) = 49.16$, $p < .001$). As shown in the previous chapter, durations did not change under levodopa ($p > .05$). However, there is a significant change in vowel duration from baseline to DBS-ON condition, as durations are on average 8 ms longer with activated DBS ($p < .001$), as the pairwise comparison revealed. This prolongation is visible across all focus types (background: +4 ms | broad: +11 ms | contrastive: +9 ms). In addition, durations in DBS-ON condition are significantly longer than durations in med-ON condition (mean difference = 10 ms, $p < .001$).

Vowel Space

VAI values remained unchanged across all conditions (med-OFF: M = 0.96, SD = 0.13 | med-ON: M = 0.95, SD = 0.08 | DBS-ON: M = 0.95, SD = 0.10), as there was no main effect of treatment ($X^2(2) = 0.2806$, $p > .05$).

9.2.3 Articulation

Figure 9.2 presents tongue body movement patterns averaged over focus types, vowels, and consonants in three treatment conditions: med-OFF (baseline), med-ON, and DBS-ON. Tongue body movements behave differently when comparing levodopa intake and activated DBS to the baseline condition. The comparison from baseline to med-ON on the left side indicates the levodopa effect. The DBS effect is presented by a comparison from baseline to DBS-ON on the right side.

The statistical analysis reveals a main effect of treatment on tongue body movement duration ($X^2(2) = 23.495$, $p < .001$). Post-hoc comparisons indicate that movement durations are shorter under levodopa ($p = .009$), as reported before in chapter 7. While durations between the baseline and the DBS-ON condition do not differ, they differ between both treatment conditions (med-OFF: M = 194, SD = 46 | med-ON: M = 187, SD = 47 | DBS-ON: M = 194, SD = 46). Movement durations are longer after activated DBS compared to levodopa intake ($p < .001$).

In addition, main effects of treatment were found on movement amplitude ($X^2(2) = 18.421$, $p < .001$) and peak velocity ($X^2(2) = 38.687$, $p < .001$). While both parameters do not change between baseline and med-ON condition, they change between baseline and DBS-ON condition. Pairwise comparisons reveal that amplitudes in DBS-ON condition are smaller compared to baseline (mean difference = -0.75 mm, $p < .001$) and to med-ON condition (mean difference = -0.5, $p = .017$). Along with this, peak velocities are slower under activated DBS (med-OFF: M = 74, SD = 41 | med-ON: M = 77, SD = 44 | DBS-ON: M = 67, SD = 40). Compared to baseline, the peak velocity is estimated to be 7 mm/s slower ($p < .001$), and compared to med-ON condition, it is estimated to be 11 mm/s slower ($p < .001$). Therefore, movement amplitudes and peak velocity reduce when DBS is activated.

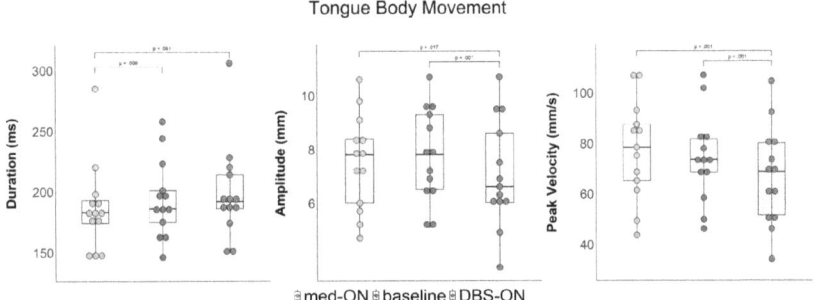

Figure 9.2. Tongue body movement patterns in relation to both treatments compared to the preoperative baseline (med-OFF). Levodopa effect: baseline to med-ON condition. DBS-effect: baseline to DBS-ON condition.

9.3 Interim Conclusion

Both treatments have shown to increase motor functions. But the improvement due to DBS tended to be smaller than that of levodopa treatment. Especially axial symptoms and symptoms related to posture and gait respond significantly less.

Intelligibility increased under both treatment conditions as well. But again, the improvement tends to be less in the case of DBS treatment. This is also indicated by the patients' self-rated speaking ability, as they

Interim Conclusion

gave themselves better ratings only after levodopa intake but not after DBS treatment.

Effects on tongue body movements differ between the treatments. While movements become shorter in med-ON condition compared to the baseline, they become slower and smaller in DBS-ON condition. In addition, acoustic vowel durations are prolonged under DBS compared to baseline. Therefore, in comparison to levodopa treatment, the speech system seems to slow down with DBS and additionally reduces in space.

The prolongation of acoustic vowel durations and the slowdown of tongue body movements cannot be explained by the DBS effect itself (cf. Chapter 8), as no change in these properties was observed comparing DBS-OFF and DBS-ON condition. Apart from speaker-specific behavior, another reason for these changes might be the influence of other factors, such as disease progression, presence of electrodes in the brain, and cognitive decline, among others things. In the next chapter I will therefore try to find an answer and explore some explanations for why speech is reduced in time and space under DBS.

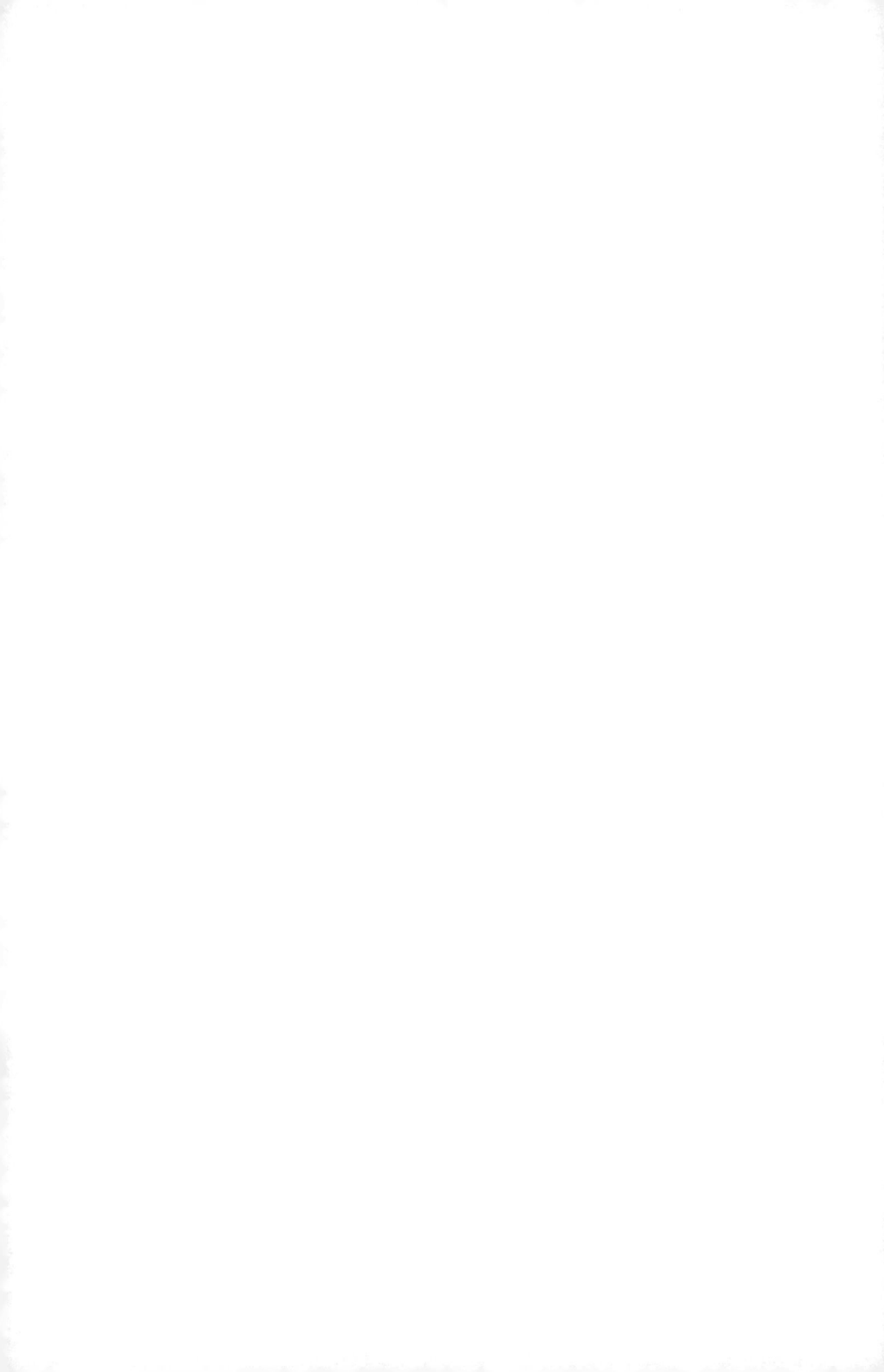

10 Results: Electrode Effect

The previous chapter showed that the effects of levodopa and STN-DBS on speech differ. Under STN-DBS, a slowing of the speech system and reduced movement amplitudes were detected. Smaller articulatory movements are expected to negatively impact speech intelligibility.

This chapter aims to explore the parameters, besides speech, that changed in individuals with PD from the preoperative (preop) to the postoperative (postop) recordings and might explain the observed effect. Therefore, changes in the neuropsychological status, disease progression, and drug reduction will be analyzed.

Moreover, it will be possible to examine the influence of the mere presence of electrodes in the brain on articulatory movements for the first time. To capture this potential effect, articulatory movements of speakers with PD are compared in the preoperative med-OFF and the postoperative DBS-OFF condition. Thus, speech patterns will be analyzed and compared without any therapeutic influences.

10.1 General Assessment

12 months (SD = 4) have elapsed between the preoperative and postoperative assessments. However, no change in neuropsychometric tests can be determined within this year. The BDI score for depression did not differ between the preoperative and postoperative assessment (preop: M = 6, SD = 4 | postop: M = 5, SD = 3). In addition, results of both tests investigating symptoms of dementia showed no change from the preoperative (MMSE: M = 28, SD = 2 | PANDA: M = 22, SD = 5) to the postoperative visit (MMSE: M = 29, SD = 1 | PANDA: M = 22, SD = 6).

In fact, individuals with PD were able to reduce drug dosages after DBS implantation. The average drug dosage was reduced by 54 % (SD = 26) from 1017 mg (SD = 290) per day to 485 mg (SD = 331) in this cohort. Of the total dose, dopamine agonists accounted for 293 mg (SD = 183) preoperatively, and 107 mg (SD = 93) postoperatively. The amount of agonists taken by patients reduced by 59 % (SD = 35) from preoperative to postoperative visit. An overview of drug dosages per patient is provided in Table A.11 in the appendix. The time from the last agonist intake to the experimental testing was the same in the preoperative and postoperative testing (preop: M = 23 hours, SD = 7 | postop: M = 24 hours, SD = 7).

Overall motor functions, measured with the UPDRS III, did not change between the preoperative med-OFF and postoperative DBS-OFF condition (med-OFF: M = 26, SD = 11 | DBS-OFF: M = 26, SD = 9). This is confirmed by the linear model (F(-1) = 0.0422, p > .05). In addition, no change was observed in the UPDRS III subscores with the exception of the PIGD score, which improved by an average of 59 % from 4 points (SD = 4) preop to 3 points (SD = 3) postop. However, as it can be seen in Figure 10.1, the UPDRS III scores develop differently across patients. Each dot represents a patient, and the treatment condition is color coded: med-OFF in pink and DBS-OFF in blue. Three patients have lower UPDRS III scores in DBS-OFF condition (7 - 8 points difference), four have higher scores (5 - 17 points difference) and five remain the same (0 - 3 points difference). One individual with PD (PD06) stands out with a strong increase of 17 points.

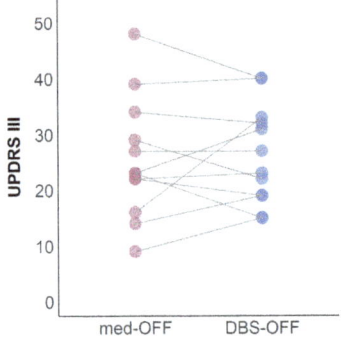

Figure 10.1. Motor scores per patient comparing preoperative med-OFF and postoperative DBS-OFF condition.

10.2 Speech Assessment

10.2.1 Speech Ratings

Intelligibility and Naturalness

In a study by Tripoliti et al. (2011), speech intelligibility was reported to deteriorate from the preoperative med-OFF condition to the postoperative med-OFF/DBS-OFF condition. In this data set, neither intelligibility (med-OFF: M = 69, SD = 26 | DBS-OFF: M = 69, SD = 26 | $\hat{\beta}$ = -0.03, p > .05) nor naturalness (med-OFF: M = 66, SD = 26 | DBS-OFF: M = 67, SD = 26 | $\hat{\beta}$ = 0.03, p > .05) changed from preoperative to postoperative OFF condition, according to the listener ratings. In both continuous ordinal regression models each rating category was taken as the dependent variable and treatment condition (med-OFF vs DBS-OFF) as predictor variable. Random intercepts were included for speaker and rater.

VAS Rating

The speakers' self-ratings on the VAS did not change from med-OFF condition to DBS-OFF condition (med-OFF: M = 7.5, SD = 2.0 | DBS-OFF: M = 5.8, SD = 3.0), as the continuous ordinal regression model reveals ($\hat{\beta}$ = 1.45, p > .05). Within the model, treatment condition was included as the predictor variable and speaker as the random intercept. However, a trend towards lower self-perceived speaking ability is visible in DBS-OFF condition.

10.2.2 Acoustics

Vowel Duration

Table 10.1 compares acoustic vowel durations averaged across vowels and consonants between med-OFF and DBS-OFF condition. Vowel durations increase from med-OFF to DBS-OFF condition. The prolongation is present in all focus conditions.

The main effects of group ($X^2(1)$ = 29.042, p < .001) and focus type ($X^2(2)$ = 23.521, p < .001) were significant. Pairwise comparisons revealed that vowel durations are longer in DBS-OFF condition compared to med-OFF condition (mean difference = 9 ms, p < .001). Moreover,

Table 10.1. Means and standard deviations of acoustic vowel durations in ms per focus type in the preoperative OFF and postoperative OFF condition.

	Vowel Duration (ms)	
	med-OFF	DBS-OFF
background	123 (34)	129 (33)
broad	132 (35)	141 (38)
contrastive	138 (36)	149 (39)
mean (sd)	131 (36)	140 (37)

prosodic adjustments were found in terms of increasing vowel durations from background to broad focus (mean difference = 11 ms, $p < .001$), from background to contrastive focus (mean difference = 18 ms, $p < .001$), and from broad to contrastive focus (mean difference = 7 ms, $p = .003$). This indicates that vowel durations are adjusted across and within accentuation.

Vowel Space

The overall vowel space exhibits small differences when comparing the VAI values in med-OFF condition (background: M = 0.93, SD = 0.13 | broad: M = 0.97, SD = 0.12 | contrastive: M = 0.97, SD = 0.14) to those in DBS-OFF condition (background: M = 0.93, SD = 0.11 | broad: M = 0.95, SD = 0.09 | contrastive: M = 0.96, SD = 0.09). There is neither a main effect of treatment condition ($X^2(1) = 0.3209$, $p > .05$) nor of focus type ($X^2(2) = 3.1722$, $p > .05$). However, the data is less variable in DBS-OFF condition and VAI values tend to be smaller.

10.2.3 Articulation

While tongue body movement durations (med-OFF: M = 195, SD = 47 | DBS-OFF: M = 194, SD = 46 | $X^2(1) = 0.0246$, $p > .05$) did not differ between both conditions, peak velocities and amplitudes did show changes. Figure 10.2 presents the results for peak velocity and amplitude data averaged across focus types, vowels, and consonants. The post-hoc comparison reveal that amplitudes decreased by 0.9 mm from preoperative to postoperative condition (med-OFF: M = 7.7, SD = 4.5 | DBS-OFF: M = 6.8, SD = 4.4 | $X^2(1) = 27.113$, $p < .001$). In addition, peak velocities were about 7 mm/s slower in DBS-OFF condition (med-OFF: M = 73, SD = 41 | DBS-OFF: M = 66, SD = 40 | $X^2(1)$ = 18.823, p < .001).

It seems that the symmetry profiles of movements in the vowels /a/ or /i/ differ between med-OFF and DBS-OFF condition and become more asymmetrical in DBS-OFF condition (Table 10.2). This is due to shorter acceleration phases that can be measured in DBS-OFF condition, particularly in the accented condition. However, no main effect of treatment condition was found ($X^2(1)$ = 1.1489, p > .05). The movements' stiffness also remains the same (med-OFF: M = 9.3, SD = 2.0 | DBS-OFF: M = 9.6, SD = 2.5 | $X^2(1)$ = 1.1884, p > .05).

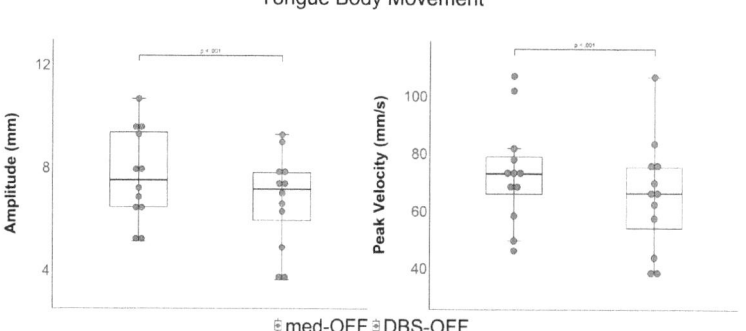

Figure 10.2. Tongue body movement amplitude and peak velocity comparing preoperative med-OFF and postoperative DBS-OFF condition.

Table 10.2. Means and standard deviations for values describing the movement profile and corresponding phases in med-OFF and DBS-OFF. ACC = acceleration phase, DEC = deceleration phase, SYMM = symmetry profile.

	med-OFF			DBS-OFF		
	ACC	DEC	SYMM	ACC	DEC	SYMM
background	94 (35)	98 (34)	1.2 (0.7)	95 (40)	97 (25)	1.2 (0.6)
broad	104 (39)	102 (35)	1.1 (0.6)	100 (39)	107 (29)	1.3 (0.7)
contrastive	100 (30)	109 (40)	1.2 (0.7)	97 (37)	111 (30)	1.3 (0.7)
mean (sd)	100 (35)	103 (36)	1.2 (0.6)	97 (39)	105 (29)	1.3 (0.7)

10.2.4 Correlation

Amplitudes and peak velocities of tongue body movements decrease from med-OFF to DBS-OFF condition. As nearly one year has passed between the preoperative and postoperative testing, it could be assumed that disease progression influences speech. As disease progression can be captured by the UPDRS III score, Figure 10.3 shows the relationship between the time elapsed between the two visits and the percentage change in the total UPDRS III score. Each dot represents one patient. Patients that are located below the gray dotted line have higher UPDRS III scores at the postoperative visit, whereas patients above the line have lower scores at that visit. The coefficient of a Pearson correlation indicates a positive relationship, suggesting that UPDRS III scores are lower when more time has passed between both OFF condition assessments ($r(10) = .53, p > .05$). This correlation is not expected, since the opposite relationship would indicate disease progression.

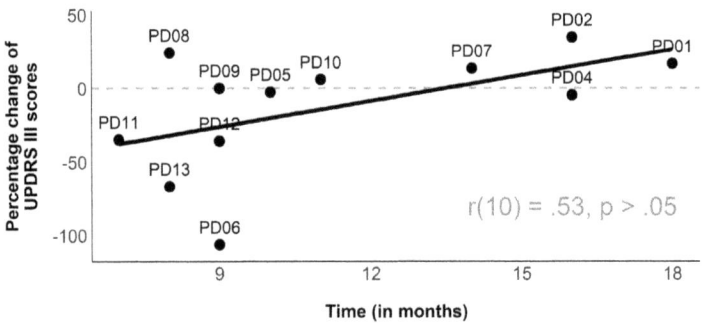

Figure 10.3. Correlation between the percentage change in motor functions and the time passed from preoperative to postoperative visit.

Another Pearson correlation reveals a positive but not significant correlation between the percentage change of UPDRS III scores and the percentage change in movement amplitude from med-OFF to DBS-OFF (Pearson: $r(10) = .34, p > .05$). This indicates larger movement amplitudes if motor impairment is more pronounced (contrary to expectations).

No relation was found between the change in axial impairment and movement amplitude (Spearman: $r(10) = -.18$, $p > .05$). In addition, the reduced amount of dopamine agonists was not shown to correlate with a change in movement amplitude (Pearson: $r(10) = -.25$, $p > .05$).

10.3 Interim Conclusion

Motor functions did not change from preoperative to postoperative visit. This indicates on average no disease progression. Moreover, no differences were noticed by naive listeners in terms of perceived intelligibility or naturalness. The speakers themselves did not perceive any differences in their speaking ability, but there is a trend towards lower self-rated speech ability after DBS implantation.

The prolonged acoustic vowel durations that can be observed in DBS-ON condition compared to med-ON condition are already present in DBS-OFF condition. In addition, the amplitude of tongue body movements tended to be reduced after DBS implantation, leading to slower movements that can be observed in DBS-OFF condition. These changes might therefore already be caused by electrode implantation and not only by activated stimulation, as none of the observed speech changes can be attributed to disease progression, cognitive decline or the amount of drugs taken.

11 Discussion

This dissertation investigated tongue body movements during vowel production in speakers with Parkinson's disease (PD) and healthy control speakers. For the first time, the same group of speakers with PD was assessed before and after the implantation of deep brain stimulation (DBS) in the nucleus subthalamicus to analyze the treatment effects of levodopa and deep brain stimulation on speech patterns. Speech was recorded with an electromagnetic articulograph to track underlying articulatory movements.

The differences between healthy control speakers and speakers with PD were explored to determine the disease effect. In addition, speech parameters were compared within the patient group to capture the treatment effect of levodopa and of DBS. The following chapter is structured in a way that allows for the results to be discussed in exactly this order. In addition, the possibility of the implantation of electrodes alone having an effect on speech will be discussed. Individual variation, compensation strategies, clinical implications, and limitations will be addressed as well.

11.1 Disease Effect

Comparing the motor results of healthy control participants and participants with PD, motor impairment was detected in individuals with PD. While axial symptoms and postural deficits were found only in the PD group, bradykinesia and rigidity were significantly more pronounced in individuals with PD compared to the healthy control group. Motor impairment is partly responsible for speech changes in individuals with PD. Axial impairment, particularly in individuals with PD, is responsible for speech deficits, as already proposed previously (Rusz, Tykalová, Novotnỳ, et al., 2021; Skodda et al., 2012). Axial symptoms are correlated with the articulation space, with the vowel articulation index (VAI) being lower when axial impairment was more pronounced. In addition, a smaller articulation space is correlated with reduced intelligibility. This evidence confirms the assumption that greater axial motor impairment is responsible for spatial reduction on the articulatory level and lower intelligibility.

In general, speech of speakers with PD was rated as less intelligible and less natural by naive listeners. This is in line with previous studies that also reported reduced intelligibility and naturalness in speakers with PD (Klopfenstein, 2016; Stipancic et al., 2016; Anand & Stepp, 2015). The patients' self-rated speaking ability, however, does not reflect this difference, as the average VAS scores were the same in both groups. It has been previously reported that individuals with PD rate themselves higher than they are rated by others (Maier & Prigatano, 2017; Leritz et al., 2004). This could explain the missing difference with regard to the ratings.

Speakers with PD in this cohort had only mild dysarthric symptoms that already seemed to affect the articulation of the tongue. This indicates further that already mild dysarthria is reflected in reduced intelligibility (Tjaden et al., 2014) and that articulation in particular has the greatest impact on intelligibility as already described in previous studies (Thies et al., 2020; Delvaux et al., 2018; Antolík & Fougeron, 2013; Skodda, Visser, & Schlegel, 2011; Kim et al., 2011). Interestingly, intelligibility is negatively correlated with longer acoustic vowel durations in the control group. Therefore, longer durational properties do not only differentiate healthy control speakers from speakers with PD, they are also the possible cause of differences in intelligibility ratings across the groups.

The main aim of this study was to detect differences in tongue body movements comparing speakers with PD and healthy control speakers. The differences were expected to be manifested in the form of smaller and slower movements in the PD group (Duffy, 2019; Kearney et al., 2017). Tongue body movement durations are longer in speakers with PD, indicating that they need more time to achieve articulatory targets. Longer movements were already described by Thompson (2018), Bandini et al. (2016) and Yunusova et al. (2008) for lips, and by Wong et al. (2011) and Yunusova et al. (2008) for the tongue. This illustrates the expected slowing down of the speech system in PD, which is also reflected in longer acoustic vowel durations. Prolongations in the temporal domain are seen as an indicator for dysarthria (Ackermann et al., 1995). In contrast to previous studies (Thies et al., 2022; Kent et al., 2000; Forrest & Weismer, 1995), prolongations were not evoked by longer deceleration phases, but by a prolongation of the entire movement. However, values of movement phases only refer to the production of the vowels /i/ and /a/ in this study. Therefore, the asymmetries found in previous studies could be driven by the inter-stage vowels /e/ and /o/, but also /u/, as these require more precise articulation to find the correct target.

With regard to changes in the spatial domain, the results are less clear. Due to the small sample size and the high individual variation, group differences reported in previous literature, such as smaller vowel spaces, were not detected. Trends in this data set point towards smaller articulation spaces but larger tongue body movement amplitudes. However, lower VAI values reflect reduced vowel contrasts and vowel centralization in the PD group. This is in line with studies showing a reduced and centralized acoustic vowel space (Hsu et al., 2017; Whitfield & Goberman, 2014; Rusz, Cmejla, Tykalová, et al., 2013; Sapir et al., 2003; Weismer et al., 2001). What is more surprising is the trend towards larger movement amplitudes, as smaller ones would have been expected within an overall reduced articulation space. However, as Wong et al. (2011) described, especially patients with dysarthric symptoms produce larger and longer tongue movements compared to healthy controls. According to this, underlying articulatory patterns are not reflected on the acoustic level. The possibility of compensation strategies to explain larger amplitudes will be discussed later on (cf. Section 11.6). In summary, assuming amplitudes of equal height in both groups, but longer movement durations in the PD group, the stiffness is reduced in speakers with PD leading to higher speaking effort.

Another question was whether timing patterns of articulatory movements would differ between the two groups. But no differences were found regarding the timing of the targets or the timing of the onsets. This indicates that this cohort of speakers with PD shows no problems with the initiation of tongue body movements. This is in line with the result of Yunusova et al. (2008) and Weismer et al. (2003), who already reported stable and preserved timing patterns. Moreover, movement phases in the production of the vowels /i/ and /a/ were comparable across the two groups. A similar observation had been made for lip movements (Kim et al., 2021). Thus, the asymmetrical movement patterns in the vowels /i/ and /a/, observed in the present study, may be related to aging and not to PD (Thies et al., 2022; Mücke et al., 2021; Hermes et al., 2018).

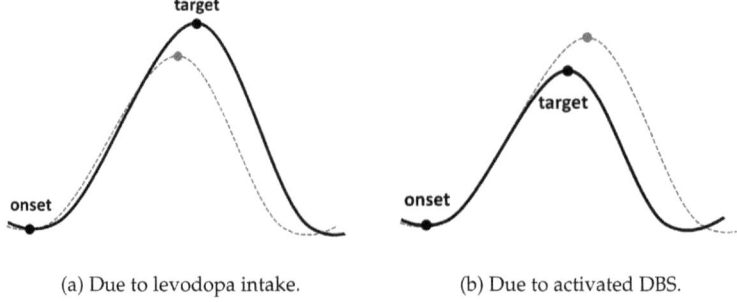

(a) Due to levodopa intake.   (b) Due to activated DBS.

Figure 11.1. Schematized treatment effects on tongue body movements.

11.2 Levodopa Effect

The intake of the controlled amount of 200 mg soluble levodopa improved motor functions in the PD group. Not only the total UPDRS III score was lower in med-ON condition, but also all motor subscores were positively impacted. This replicates the effect of levodopa intake on gross motor functions. In contrast to some other findings, axial symptoms improved by the same percentage as overall motor functions (Kalia & Lang, 2015).

While motor symptoms of all speakers with PD improved and changed in the same direction, speech pattern responded differently. The heterogeneity of speech patterns explains why the research situation is rather opaque. The present study did only find significant differences in the temporal domain, as tongue body movement durations are shorter under levodopa. However, trends are observable in the spatial domain. Parameters in the spatial domain change on average towards a reduced articulation space, as reported by Martel Sauvageau et al. (2015), and smaller movement amplitudes. However, these trends, referring only to mean values, are misleading, as only a few speakers shift the data distribution in this direction. The majority of speakers enhance the entire articulatory movement by producing longer, larger, and faster movements after levodopa intake (Figure 11.1a).

The lack of significant speech effects is not due to the fact that nothing changes after levodopa intake, but rather a consequence of speakers behaving differently. The data is highly variable and causes uncertainty in the statistical analysis, which does not reveal a clear levodopa effect. Most of the speakers with PD change speech parameters in both temporal and spatial dimensions, combining different modification strategies. The most frequent strategy is the combination of a target overshoot and a rescaling of the entire movement. Six patients showed longer, larger, and faster tongue body movements in med-ON condition. This indicates a more agile tongue body that is able to articulate more precisely (hyper-articulation). An enhancement of tongue body movements further increases intelligibility, which is beneficial to speech perception. Another strategy is the combination of a target undershoot and a shrinking of the entire movement, leading to shorter, smaller, and slower movements in three speakers with PD. This also reflects an increase in the tongue body agility and a more efficient speech production (hypo-articulation). Both strategies indicate a beneficial effect of levodopa on the speech motor function.

Apart from this, stable timing pattern of articulatory targets were observed in both treatment conditions. Vocalic targets were stably achieved within 69 % of the acoustic syllable. This is in line with findings of Thies et al. (2022, 2021). The data reveals further that the onset is initiated later in med-ON condition, indicating improved speech planning skills in terms of tongue body movement initiation, as the distance between the articulatory onset and the acoustic syllable start is reduced. This effect was reported previously (Thies et al., 2021).

With regard to intelligibility and naturalness, the speech output is rated more intelligible under levodopa, while naturalness ratings did not change. Thus, improved motor functions are reflected in particular in more intelligible speech under levodopa. This improvement is also noticed by the patients themselves and is probably due to improved axial symptoms.

11.3 DBS Effect

Clear evidence for how deep brain stimulation influences speech is still lacking. This is mainly due to the fact that the methodology of previous studies varies greatly. Especially studies that investigated the influence of deep brain stimulation on speech under regular medication were not able to analyze the influence of each treatment individually.

The present study investigated the pure effect of STN-DBS on speech. However, no significant differences between DBS-OFF and DBS-ON condition were found. This is not due to the fact that no changes were observed after activating DBS, but rather a consequence of speaker-specific behavior. Most of the speakers showed smaller movement amplitudes under activated DBS (hypo-articulation; Figure 11.1b), indicating lower speech effort on the one hand, but less distinct articulation on the other hand. Six speakers with PD rescaled tongue body movements under activated DBS, resulting in shorter and smaller movements. This indicates a shrinking of the whole movement pattern. Two others presented smaller and shorter or only smaller tongue body movements respectively. In contrast, three speakers with PD rescaled tongue body movements in the opposite direction by enhancing them in each domain (longer and larger movements). The more widely used hypo-articulation in DBS-ON condition can be related to more efficient speech production on the one hand, but also to a reduced flexibility in time and space on the other hand. While the first explanation indicates a beneficial effect of DBS, the latter would be an aggravation. The tendency points towards a reduced spatial modulation, as spatial adjustments were also no longer used as a strategy for prominence marking.

In line with previous research, motor functions improved by 50 % under DBS. Improvement is attributed in particular to changes in rigidity and bradykinesia. Subscores related to axial symptoms and gait and posture did not change and can be considered stimulation-refractory (Lozano et al., 2019; Benabid, 2003). Fabbri et al. (2017) concluded that speech behaves similar to gait and posture. As VAI values correlated with axial motor symptoms and PIGD subscores in the present study, this could explain why the acoustic vowel space did not change under DBS.

The results highlight that speech and motor functions do not respond in a similar way. Moreover, response patterns concerning speech differ between levodopa intake and activated DBS. Thus, the implantation of DBS electrodes appears to change speech patterns. This will be discussed in the following section.

11.4 Electrode Effect

Another surprising finding of this thesis is that the mere presence of electrodes in the brain may lead to smaller and slower tongue body movements. The first assumption to explain this result is that the disease continues to progress between the preoperative and the postoperative visit. But motor skills remained on average on the same level. One exception is patient PD06, whose UPDRS III scores immensely increased. This poses the question of whether patients who produce smaller amplitudes have higher UPDRS III total scores and/or greater axial impairment. Interestingly, tongue body amplitudes seem to be larger when motor impairment is more pronounced. This behavior contradicts expectations, but it highlights a possible compensation strategy that will be discussed in detail later on (cf. Section 11.6).

A micro lesion effect that refers to the impact of electrode implantation immediately after surgery can also be excluded. On the one hand, no clear motor improvement was observed, as reported in other studies (Mestre et al., 2016; Cersosimo et al., 2009), that is further reflected in speech patterns. On the other hand, testing was carried out at least five months after surgery ensuring that edema are resolved and the stimulation effect is stabilized (Mestre et al., 2016; Castrioto et al., 2013; Kern & Kumar, 2007). However, due to chronic stimulation of the brain areas within and around the STN for at least five months, neural networks may have reorganized. The resulting new connections might stay functional even if the stimulation is switched off for a short amount of time. This neuroplasticity might cause a deterioration of speech and lead to smaller movements, as found in this study. Structural changes in patients with PD as a result of long-term STN-DBS were reported previously by van Hartevelt et al. (2014). Interestingly, those patients who have had DBS electrodes implanted for more than a year present with lower UPDRS III scores in DBS-OFF. Their motor functions show improvement, which runs counter to the idea of disease progression.

Another explanation could be poorly implanted electrodes. But as it can be seen in Figure 5.1, electrodes were successfully implanted and well positioned in the dorsolateral STN without causing lesions to the caudate nucleus. Per in-house protocols, the caudate nucleus is avoided during stereotactic planning to limit the detrimental effect of DBS on cognitive abilities (Witt et al., 2013). In accordance with these precautions, the patients' cognitive skills did not change from the preoperative to the postoperative visit.

It is well known that patients can reduce the daily amount of drugs after DBS implantation. This is also mirrored in the present study, as patients reduced the levodopa equivalent daily dosage by about 54 % and the amount of agonists by 59 %. Therefore, the drug reduction in this cohort of individuals with PD is rather high (Liang et al., 2006; Rodriguez-Oroz et al., 2005; Benabid, 2003). As dopamine agonists have a longer plasma half-life than levodopa (Reichmann, 2009), the reduction of agonists might explain the resulting reduced movement amplitudes at the postoperative visit. The higher the amount of agonists acting in the body, the more durable the effect on motor functions. Accordingly, speech functions may benefit longer before surgery than after surgery, when fewer agonists are taken, although medications were suspended. However, neither the time since the last agonists were taken before the experimental testing, nor the amount of agonists have been found to correlate with the speech results. Therefore, the speech changes are not related to changes of the total drug dosages or dopamine agonists. Thus, the influence of drugs can be excluded.

As argued above, changes in tongue body movement amplitudes are independent of the micro lesion effect, agonists, and disease progression. Speech changes between the preoperative med-OFF and postoperative DBS-OFF status were also reported in previous research. Tripoliti et al. (2011) reported lower intelligibility, while Robertson et al. (2011) found slower jaw movements. In this data set reduced movement amplitudes with accompanying slowness were observed. This means that the speech system was scaled down after DBS implantation and that a new starting point is defined from which DBS treatment functions.

The changes in movement amplitude seem to be too subtle to be reflected in the acoustics or the perception, since neither the VAI values nor the ratings of intelligibility or naturalness had changed. However, a trend towards lower self-perceived speaking ability is visible in DBS-OFF condition, indicating that the individuals with PD might recognize changes in tongue body movements. Reduced tongue body movements that need to be enhanced in the spatial domain for the sake of intelligibility increase the required speech effort. Therefore, the lower self-rated speaking ability of the patients reflects these higher demands after DBS implantation.

11.5 Prominence Marking

Prosodic prominence marking was investigated to analyze whether speakers with PD are capable of adjusting speech parameters according to the demands of natural communication processes. In order to challenge the flexibility of the speech system in speakers with PD, a speech production task was designed to collect speech in three different focus conditions. The investigation of prominence marking strategies was taken into account to determine if speakers with PD make use of the continuum from hypo- to hyper-articulated speech. Hypo-articulation is expected for the production of out-of-focus constituents, and hyper-articulation for the production of in-focus ones, such as broad and contrastive focus. The question was whether strategies in the PD group differ from healthy controls and change due to therapy options.

When comparing healthy control speakers and individuals with PD, while being off PD medication, speakers of both groups adjusted speech parameters on the temporal and spatial domain to express prosodic prominence. Previous research reported that speakers with PD do mark prominence, but not as effectively as healthy controls, and that strategies vary (Thies et al., 2020; Tykalová et al., 2014; Azevedo et al., 2013; Cheang & Pell, 2007). So the assumption was that speakers with PD would adjust prosodic speech parameters across accentuation (unaccented vs. accented condition) but not within accentuation (broad focus vs. contrastive focus).

Both groups adjusted temporal and spatial parameters only across accentuation. Since longer durations are perceptually associated with an increase in sonority, both groups made use of the sonority expansion strategy by increasing acoustic vowel and tongue body movement durations under prominence (De Jong et al., 1993; Beckman et al., 1992). With respect to the spatial domain, both groups showed more extreme tongue positions under prominence. Larger displacements are associated with the production of more peripheral vowels with the aim of enhancing prosodic contrasts, indicating that the hyper-articulation strategy is also applied (Mücke & Grice, 2014; Harrington et al., 2000; De Jong, 1995). As movement amplitudes and the respective acoustic vowel space are only adjusted across accentuation, they do not express different degrees of prosodic prominence within accentuation. This behavior was already suggested in the recent literature (Roessig et al., 2022). As articulatory features are already enhanced in the broad focus condition, there is no space left to adjust articulation further to the periphery for contrastive focus production. However, speakers with PD descriptively showed more fine-grained adjustments on the spatial level, as they increased acoustic vowel space across and within accentuation, while healthy controls only adjusted it across accentuation. This differentiation comes at the expense of a greater speech effort in the spatial domain to express prominence. In sum, the results suggest that speakers with PD preserve linguistic function in important positions, if required (Antolík & Fougeron, 2013; Ackermann & Ziegler, 1991).

Another question is whether prominence-marking strategies differ between treatment conditions. When comparing prosodic adjustments in med-OFF and med-ON condition, the adjustments observed are more fine-grained and efficient under levodopa. For example, the acoustic vowel space was enhanced equally to all sides, while a strong retraction of the vowels /u/ and /o/ was observed in med-OFF condition. Moreover, speakers with PD increased acoustic vowel durations not only across but also within accentuation. Improved prosodic control contradicts with the findings of Elfmarková et al. (2016), who assumed that prosodic features might not be controlled by dopaminergic circuits. However, phonatory parameters were investigated in the study, suggesting that the articulatory system should be considered separately from the phonatory system in terms of levodopa response. Prominence strategies did also change after DBS implantation. Acoustic vowel durations were adjusted across and within accentuation, while tongue movement amplitudes were only modulated across accentuation. Temporal modulations were stronger than before surgery and might compensate for less flexible spatial adjustments that are caused by the electrodes in the brain. However, both treatments increase the ability to apply prosodic-marking strategies on the temporal level.

To sum up, the data reveal that tongue body movements become larger and longer under prominence in speakers with PD, supporting the results that prosodic marking is maintained on the articulatory level in PD (Kim et al., 2021). As an increase in duration and amplitude is associated with an increase in prominence (Katsika, 2018; Mücke & Grice, 2014; Cho, 2006), speakers with PD make use of sonority-expansion and hyper-articulation strategies. So far, the role of peak velocity can be described as inconclusive based on previous literature (Pagel et al., 2020). According to this data set, peak velocity does not play a role in prominence marking. This suggests that movements are rescaled for prominence marking in general.

11.6 Compensation Strategies

Compensation strategies appear to counteract effects of aging, dysarthria or motor impairment as well as delayed auditory feedback.

The large degree of variation in the data regarding the spatial domain explains the lack of a significant difference and certainty in the output of the fitted linear mixed models. In both groups, some speakers showed smaller and some larger movement amplitudes. Those that produce larger amplitudes might be in a compensation phase characterized by hyper-articulation. This is the case for speakers aged 55 to 59, as they might compensate for aging effects (PD11, PD12, CON04, CON11; Schreen, Thies, Hermes, & Mücke, 2022). In the case of speakers with PD in particular, it might be a combined compensation for aging and disease effects. Hyper-articulation within an overall reduced articulation space is not expected in the first place. However, articulatory movements of speakers with mild dysarthria were previously observed to be larger compared to those in healthy control speakers (Wong et al., 2011). This target overshoot can function as a compensatory strategy to counteract disease effects, as larger amplitudes correlated with greater motor impairment. Another idea is that speakers with PD counteract phonatory decline as hypokinetic dysarthria in PD appears to start with phonatory deficits and evolves towards articulatory deficits. A study by Mefferd and Dietrich (2019) observed larger tongue movements in a speaker group that only had phonatory-prosodic deficits, while the group that had additional articulatory deficits tended to have smaller amplitudes. In this case, hyper-articulation would counteract hypo-adduction of the vocal folds that leads to the characteristic harsh and breathy voice quality in PD.

Speakers may maintain this compensatory behavior for a while until influences of the disease or the severity of the dysarthria become too dominant. The speech system will then change towards hypo-articulation, articulatory undershoot and an overall reduced articulation space, as seen in speakers PD01 and PD02. These speakers with PD show small movement amplitudes and cannot compensate any longer, as the dysarthric symptoms affecting the tongue have become more severe or because their deficits regarding motor performance are too pronounced. Thus, the typical features of a hypokinetic dysarthria are present at this stage. This reveals that some speakers of this cohort are located more on the left end and some more on the right end of the hyper-, hypo-continuum (independent of prominence marking), indicating different stages of adaptation as proposed by Brunner et al. (2006).

Target overshoot or prolongations could also be seen as strategies to compensate for delayed auditory feedback (Brendel et al., 2004; Rousseau & Watts, 2002; Yorkston et al., 1999). As speech production in speakers with PD is slowed down, this may support feedback control in speakers with PD to reach the articulatory target at the right time (Thies et al., 2022; Mücke et al., 2021; Hermes et al., 2018; Ostry et al., 1987). In this respect, longer deceleration phases were expected in speakers with PD, but they did not differ between the groups or treatment conditions. The specific phases of acceleration and deceleration are longer in speakers with PD, but proportionally stable and comparable to healthy control speakers. Thus, this asymmetry is presumably related to aging rather than the disease as far as the vowels /i/ and /a/ are concerned (Thies et al., 2022). PD could therefore rather influence the vowels /e/ and /o/, which do not have a clear articulatory target like wide open or fully closed, but are situated in the inter-staged articulation space.

In addition, this study revealed not only different strategies in connection to Parkinson's disease itself but also to treatment options. Most speakers with PD make use of rescaling strategies by either enhancing tongue body movements or reducing them as consequence of treatment. Duffy (2019) described that individuals with PD have scaling problems with regard to amplitude and duration. In response to levodopa intake many speakers hyper-articulate. This behavior is reflected in longer and larger movements that should also reduce the movements' stiffness and increase the speech effort. In contrast, DBS treatment leads to shorter, smaller, and stiffer movements (hypo-articulation). In general, speakers strive for a balanced cost-benefit ratio (McGuire & Botvinick, 2010; Lindblom, 1990). Hyper-articulation is associated with higher effort and therefore higher costs. After levodopa intake speakers make a greater speech effort by producing longer and larger tongue body movements. In contrast, the speech effort is smaller in DBS-ON condition, as movements are shorter and smaller. The reduction in space is accompanied by a reduction in intelligibility in DBS-ON condition (Tsuboi et al., 2015). This points towards less distinct articulation and the articulatory goal not being fully reached.

11.7 Variation

The data indicate the expected stable target alignment in all conditions, which reflects goal-directed speech production. Thus, the vocalic target functions as an anchor for goal-directed tongue body movements. However, in contrast to consonantal movements, vocalic movements allow for much variation and for targets to be achieved in different ways (Perrier & Fuchs, 2015). The excess degrees of freedom of the articulatory system, as described by Löfqvist (2010), might also explain why the articulatory results are not reflected in the acoustics and why the articulatory-acoustic relationship is not as strong as indicated by Mefferd (2015). For example, in smaller articulation spaces, movement amplitudes can be large, such as in PD11. The opposite case is observable for PD02, as he shows a larger articulation space, but smaller movement amplitudes.

In line with this, previous acoustic studies reported heterogeneous results for the acoustic level and the articulatory level (Fivela et al., 2014; Dromey & Bjarnason, 2011; Pinto et al., 2005). A lot of speaker-specific variation is visible in the data and it is even higher in the PD group than in the control group. Although variability is natural, especially in the production of vowels, it complicates the characterization of movement patterns. Due to a few speakers showing very strong changes, the data distribution is shifted into a direction that no longer reflects the behavior of the majority. In this sense, the averages indicate shorter movement durations under levodopa, although most speakers have longer ones. For activated DBS, the opposite is true, as the means indicate increased movement durations, while most patients shorten them.

For example, speaker PD11 produced much longer durations in all conditions compared to the other speakers. This reflects this subjects' low speech tempo and observed dysfluencies that were assessed by a speech pathologist. He has the highest intelligibility ratings but the lowest naturalness ratings. Due to levodopa intake, already long and large movements are further increased in time and enhanced in space. DBS leads to modulations in only the temporal domain, leading to even longer movements. These patterns differ from the rest of the group. Under DBS he presents with longer, smaller, and slower tongue body movements compared to DBS-OFF condition. As Wong et al. (2011) described, a combination of these characteristics was found in speakers without dysarthria. For this speaker it might indicate rather an improvement of articulatory deficits, as a dysarthria is certainly present but intelligibility maintained.

In addition, it should be mentioned that some speakers respond in the same way to levodopa and DBS treatment, while others change their patterns. For example, PD01 has reduced amplitudes in the OFF conditions that become even smaller in the ON conditions. Conversely, speaker PD12 has larger amplitudes than the rest of the PD group and produces even larger ones under both treatments. However, movement velocity responds differently, as his movements become faster under levodopa and slower with DBS. In contrast, PD02 basically shows smaller and slower movements that become smaller and slower under levodopa, but larger and faster with activated DBS. This observation indicates that strategies are not maintained per speaker and are not speaker- or treatment-specific.

Reasons for speaker-specific behavior can relate to disease severity, severity of dysarthria, tongue-specific impairment, as indicated by Mefferd and Dietrich (2019), and varying stimulation settings. One example for disease severity in the form of pronounced axial symptoms is PD01. He has the greatest axial impairment and produced the smallest movement amplitudes. Moreover, high-frequency stimulation is known to reduce articulatory control (Morello et al., 2020; Phokaewvarangkul et al., 2019). Two patients in this cohort do have higher stimulation frequencies compared to all other individuals with PD. PD07 is stimulated with a frequency of 174 Hz in the left hemisphere, and PD08 with a frequency of 198 Hz in both hemispheres (Table A.1). When examining the response of these two speakers to DBS treatment, it becomes apparent that their movements become shorter, smaller and slower. Especially smaller movements reveal imprecise articulation that is less distinct. In this regard, unilateral left STN was shown to reduce prosodic adjustments and articulatory precision (Wang et al., 2006; Santens et al., 2003). Therefore, high-frequency stimulation in the left STN should be avoided.

11.8 Clinical Implications

Clinical implications of this study are presented with regard to whether levodopa or DBS treatment is superior and in light of the management of the disease with respect to speech therapy.

With respect to motor functions, levodopa and DBS lead to improved overall motor skills. However, axial symptoms and those related to gait and postural instability do respond to levodopa intake but not to activated DBS. The lack of response of DBS to axial symptoms can be a challenge because the data shows that it is important to treat axial symptoms as effectively as possible to achieve the most intelligible speech output. Accordingly, the best possible improvement of axial symptoms should be aimed for. Furthermore, as discussed above, high-frequency stimulation in the left STN should be avoided.

When comparing the levodopa and DBS effect on speech, response patterns differ but intelligibility improves as a consequence of both treatments. While levodopa treatment leads to longer and larger tongue body movements, STN-DBS leads to shorter and smaller movements for the majority of patients. Patients hyper-articulate after levodopa intake, while they hypo-articulate when the stimulation is turned on. Hypo-articulation under DBS indicates less distinct articulation that explains why the improvement in perceived intelligibility is lower compared to levodopa treatment. Hyper-articulation increases the speech effort but also the intelligibility. Thus, patients with PD that are treated with DBS should be trained towards hyper-articulation strategies to improve their speech output.

The common goal of speech therapy is to increase speech intelligibility. According to the data presented in this study, a higher vowel articulation index as a measure of the articulation space has a favorable effect on intelligibility and additionally on perceived naturalness. This indicates that larger articulation spaces should be targeted in speech therapy. Therefore, the goal of therapeutic interventions should be to increase tongue body movement amplitudes and the overall articulation space for the sake of naturalness and intelligibility gains in speakers with PD. An increase in tongue movement amplitudes and acoustic vowel contrasts is associated with clear and especially slow speech (Mefferd, 2017; Fletcher et al., 2015; Tjaden et al., 2013; McRae et al., 2002). The question, however, is how slow the speech tempo may become before the speech output becomes too unnatural, since longer durations improve intelligibility but reduce naturalness in healthy speech. This highlights the challenge of speaking intelligible and natural at the same time. Therefore, a good balance between intelligibility and naturalness should be aimed for, so that the patients speak comprehensively but not too unnatural to avoid a negative impact on their ability to communicate and participate in daily life.

11.9 Limitations

This study was exploratory in nature. Although the number of subjects is comparable to that of previous articulatory studies, it was too small to describe significant effects for most parameters, given the high variation in the data. Group or treatment effects leveled out because of speaker-specific behavior. The sample size was too small to capture clear treatment effects and to divide speakers into clusters based on heterogeneous response patterns. Future research should seek for a way to deal with outliers and for higher sample sizes to be able to determine reasons for varying speech patterns. A study by Thies et al. (2021) was able to provide significant effects of levodopa treatment with a cohort of 16 speakers with PD, reporting shorter, larger and faster tongue body movements after levodopa intake. Less variation, reduced uncertainty and significant effects can therefore be expected if the sample size is increased by a few speakers. Variability could also potentially be reduced if repetitions are included. In this study repetitions were avoided in order not to prolong the duration of the experiment in consideration of the patients' condition.

With regard to articulatory data it will be fruitful to also analyze the horizontal movement dimension in order to inspect tongue configuration difficulties in this domain, which have already been described by Weismer et al. (2012). As reported by Thies et al. (2020) and Rusz, Cmejla, Tykalová, et al. (2013), a more centralized production of the vowels /u/ and /o/ was observed. In this data set, these two vowels were strongly retracted in med-OFF condition. It is important to find out why these two vowels in particular deviate to such an extent. Therefore, in a future analysis, each vowel should be looked at individually. In a further step, an analysis strategy should be implemented for how to deal with multiple velocity peaks in order to investigate the movement phases of the vowels /e/, /o/ and /u/. As movement phases were stable and comparable across groups and conditions in this study for the vowels /i/ and /a/, deviations are presumably more likely to occur with inter-staged vowels that do not have a clearly defined articulatory target.

It also became apparent that traditional modification strategies cannot account for all changes that appear in speakers with PD. Speakers adjust speech parameters in both domains of time and space and combine traditional strategies. This indicates that the task-dynamic parameters are too simple to describe impaired speech in its entirety. Since the task-dynamic model does not consider the jaw as an independent articulator, its movements were not tracked. However, jaw movements could be analyzed more specifically in the future to examine whether jaw and tongue movements are decoupled in speech of speakers with PD (Mefferd, 2017; Henriques & van Lieshout, 2013). It could also be interesting to analyze consonantal movements in a next step. Consonantal movements are faster by nature and allow for less variation. Presumably, movement patterns differ from vocalic movements.

Another issue that can hardly be avoided is the fact that the recordings were made in an experimental setting. Lab-based performances may not be indicative of the patients' everyday way of speaking. Especially larger movements in speakers with PD compared to healthy controls could be explained in terms of motivation. Recordings were first made in med-OFF condition, so that participants' motivation might have been higher than in the proceeding recording sessions. Increasing attention and effort can lead to larger amplitudes during speech production (Obeso et al., 2014).

Despite a reduced articulation space, patients do have a motor reserve that they can retrieve if they want to improve speech performance in contrast to daily life conversations. If speakers are explicitly asked to do something, their performances improve (Kwan & Whitehill, 2011; Dromey & Adams, 2000). However, larger amplitudes are related to clear speech and hyper-articulation, which requires a higher speech effort. Increasing the speech effort is most often avoided to reduce costs if possible.

In this regard, high-costs strategies after levodopa intake in the form of longer and larger movements (hyper-articulation) could also have been evoked by an enhanced activity in the direct pathway based on the use of more dopamine than necessary. Patients received a supra-maximal dosage of levodopa that could have been too high for those individuals showing these speech patterns. Therefore, the study protocol could be repeated with individual dosages.

To answer the question of whether hyper-articulation is a compensation strategy in earlier stages of a developing dysarthria, speech could be investigated in individuals with PD that have a moderate and severe dysarthria. In the present study, a cohort of patients with only a mild form of dysarthria have been investigated. Additionally, it would be interesting to collect data from a group treated only medically to capture speech changes over a period of one year without the implantation effect of DBS. As it was not possible to fully explain the effect of the mere presence of DBS electrodes, an idea for future work would be to investigate effects of neuroplasticity on speech. However, this is difficult to implement because DBS would need to stay deactivated for several days, not just minutes or hours, which most patients will not tolerate. Another idea would be to resort to imaging data, as was done by Wirsching et al. (2018) and van Hartevelt et al. (2014).

12 Conclusion

This work has provided insights into speech changes related to Parkinson's disease, levodopa intake and deep brain stimulation (DBS). Three levels related to speech production were investigated in speakers with PD: kinematics, acoustics and perception.

Speech of speakers with PD is less intelligible compared to healthy controls but intelligibility increases with levodopa and DBS treatment. Individuals with PD are aware of speech changes that increase intelligibility, as they rate their speaking ability higher in therapeutic conditions. To improve intelligibility, clinical management should aim for low axial impairment and a clear and slow speaking style in individuals with PD suffering from dysarthric speech.

Speakers with PD present a slowed speech system and a tendency towards smaller articulation spaces compared to healthy control speakers. The adjustments of the speech system in articulatory movements related to vowel production differ depending on the applied medical treatment. After levodopa intake, the speech effort of most speakers with PD is higher because they hyper-articulate to compensate for the limitations of the speech motor system caused by the disease. This is indicated by longer and larger movements and a more distinct articulation space. With activated DBS, speakers with PD hypo-articulate by producing shorter and smaller movements and by reducing their speech effort. Thus, speech production is reduced particularly in the spatial domain but might become more efficient to compensate for the influence of the disease. With regard to speech perception, levodopa treatment is favored, making articulation more distinct and intelligible. Although the treatment methods have different effects, the success of the therapy should be emphasized. The tongue body is more agile under levodopa and more efficient under DBS.

Speakers with PD are also able to adjust speech movements in the context of prosodic marking. Regardless of treatment condition, tongue body movements increase in duration and amplitude during vowel production in accented syllables as prominence increases. Temporal adjustments are more fine-grained when expressing different degrees of prominence, i.e., differentiating between broad focus and contrastive focus, in both therapeutic conditions.

The results indicate that speakers with PD are able to adapt to external and internal influences on the speech motor system. Thus, the speech system of mild dysarthric speakers with PD is flexible enough to control speech parameters in time and space to maintain goal-directed speech production.

Appendix

A.1 Stimulation Parameters

The following Table A.1 summarizes the stimulation parameters per patient. Information about activated contacts, pulse width, frequency, and milliampere (mA) are given for each hemisphere separately.

Table A.1. Individual stimulation settings.

Patient	Left hemisphere				Right hemisphere			
	contacts	pulse	frequency	mA	contacts	pulse	frequency	mA
PD01	5, 6, 7, 8	60	130	3.1	13, 14, 15	60	130	2.2
PD02	7, 8	60	130	1.2	3, 5, 6, 8	60	130	1.4
PD03	5, 6, 7	40	130	3.4	13, 14, 15	40	130	3.7
PD04	3, 1	60	130	2.4	13, 14, 15	60	130	0.6
PD05	2, 3, 4	60	130	0.6	2, 3, 4	60	130	0.5
PD06	2, 3, 4	60	130	0.5	2, 3, 4	60	130	0.5
PD07	5, 6, 7	60	174	2.0	5, 6, 7	60	130	0.3
PD08	5, 6, 7	30	198	1.9	5, 6, 7	30	198	2.4
PD09	2, 3, 4	60	130	3.3	5, 6, 7	60	130	1.9
PD10	5, 6, 7	60	130	1.9	5, 6, 7	60	130	1.9
PD11	2, 3, 4	60	130	0.9	2, 3, 4	60	130	0.9
PD12	5, 6, 7	60	130	2.5	7	60	130	2.3
PD13	5, 6, 7	60	130	1.8	13, 14, 15	60	130	1.8

A.2 Neuropsychological Assessment

Within this section an overview is given over neuropsychological test results. Values are reported for healthy controls (CON) and for individuals with PD at two time points: preoperative visit and postoperative visit.

Test results of the Beck-Depression-Inventory-II (BDI), the Parkinson Neuropsychometric Dementia Assessment (PANDA), and the Mini-Mental State Examination (MMSE) are provided.

Table A.2. Assessments scores of Beck-Depression-Inventory-II.

	BDI	
CON	PD - preop	PD - postop
7	0	5
0	6	3
1	11	7
0	6	8
0	3	8
0	0	5
0	9	10
0	5	3
2	10	-
7	3	3
0	4	7
0	12	2
5	8	3
mean (sd) 2 (3)	6 (4)	5 (3)

Table A.3. Results of the Parkinson Neuropsychometric Dementia Assessment.

	CON	PANDA PD - preop	PD - postop
	17	23	14
	29	30	28
	20	23	18
	30	22	14
	18	24	22
	30	14	18
	26	14	19
	19	27	17
	27	29	-
	27	24	25
	26	20	28
	22	14	21
	24	26	30
mean (sd)	24 (5)	22 (5)	22 (6)

Table A.4. Results of the Mini-Mental State Examination.

	CON	MMSE PD - preop	PD - postop
	28	24	28
	29	30	30
	29	29	30
	29	29	29
	28	29	30
	28	24	26
	28	28	29
	29	29	30
	28	29	29
	30	30	30
	30	30	30
	29	27	28
	30	29	30
mean (sd)	29 (1)	28 (2)	29 (1)

A.3 Characteristics of Dysarthria

The following Table A.5 shows for each patient which speech domain exhibits already deviations according to the mild hypokinetic dysarthria that were diagnosed by a speech pathologist.

Table A.5. Composition of dysarthric symptoms per individual with PD.

Voice quality	Speech tempo	Articulation	Prosody	Dysfluency
PD01		PD01	PD01	PD01
PD02			PD02	
	PD03	PD03		
	PD04	PD04	PD04	PD04
PD05	PD05		PD05	
PD06		PD06		
	PD07	PD07	PD07	
	PD08			
PD09				
PD10		PD10	PD10	
	PD11		PD11	PD11
PD12	PD12	PD12	PD12	
		PD13		

A.4 Results Motor Assessment

In the following, an overview over results of the motor assessment is given. Results are presented for the healthy control group and for the individuals with PD in each condition their were tested in. The total UPDRS III score and several subscores are presented. The speech score refers to item 18 of the UPDRS, axial symptoms to the sum of item 18 + items 27 to 30, bradykinesia to items 23 to 26 + item 31, rigidity to item 22, tremor to item 20 + item 21, and postural instability and gait disorder (PIGD) to items 27 to 30.

Table A.6. Overview over the scores of the motor assessment of healthy control participants based on the UPDRS III.

	total	speech	axial	bradykinesia	rigidity	tremor	PIGD
CON01	13	0	0	6	6	1	1
CON02	3	0	0	1	2	0	0
CON03	5	0	0	2	3	0	0
CON04	1	0	0	0	1	0	0
CON05	6	0	0	2	2	2	0
CON06	5	0	0	5	0	0	0
CON07	7	0	0	2	5	0	1
CON08	2	0	0	0	2	0	0
CON09	5	0	0	2	3	0	0
CON10	0	0	0	0	0	0	0
CON11	1	0	0	0	1	0	0
CON12	6	0	1	0	4	0	1
CON13	-	-	-	-	-	-	-
mean (sd)	4 (3)	0 (0)	0 (0)	2 (2)	2 (2)	0 (1)	0 (0)

Table A.7. Overview over the scores of the motor assessment of individuals with PD in med-OFF condition.

	total	speech	axial	bradykinesia	rigidity	tremor	PIGD
PD01	48	1	14	20	13	1	15
PD02	23	1	1	4	8	9	0
PD03	15	0	2	4	8	0	3
PD04	22	1	6	8	6	0	6
PD05	39	2	6	22	4	5	5
PD06	16	2	2	9	4	0	1
PD07	22	1	4	10	3	4	5
PD08	29	1	2	15	8	3	2
PD09	27	2	5	10	8	2	4
PD10	34	1	2	19	10	1	4
PD11	23	1	5	8	3	6	4
PD12	14	1	2	4	7	0	2
PD13	9	1	2	0	5	2	1
mean (sd)	25 (11)	1 (1)	4 (3)	10 (7)	7 (3)	3 (3)	4 (4)

Table A.8. Overview over the scores of the motor assessment of individuals with PD in med-ON condition.

	total	speech	axial	bradykinesia	rigidity	tremor	PIGD
PD01	17	1	7	4	5	0	6
PD02	12	0	1	1	4	5	1
PD03	12	0	0	5	5	1	0
PD04	6	0	1	3	1	0	2
PD05	6	0	1	3	1	0	1
PD06	12	2	2	7	2	0	2
PD07	7	0	1	3	1	2	2
PD08	14	1	1	8	5	0	1
PD09	14	1	3	4	6	0	2
PD10	19	1	1	7	7	3	1
PD11	7	0	0	3	1	2	0
PD12	9	2	3	2	3	0	2
PD13	9	1	1	4	3	1	0
mean (sd)	14 (9)	1 (1)	2 (2)	4 (2)	3 (2)	1 (2)	2 (2)

Results Motor Assessment

Table A.9. Overview over the scores of the motor assessment of individuals with PD in DBS-OFF condition.

	total	speech	axial	bradykinesia	rigidity	tremor	PIGD
PD01	40	2	7	17	14	0	6
PD02	15	1	2	7	0	4	1
PD03	-	-	-	-	-	-	-
PD04	23	1	2	10	8	1	1
PD05	40	3	6	18	6	8	5
PD06	33	2	9	17	5	0	10
PD07	19	1	2	6	8	2	2
PD08	22	0	1	13	5	3	2
PD09	27	1	4	11	10	1	4
PD10	32	1	3	16	8	3	4
PD11	31	2	6	10	6	8	4
PD12	19	2	3	7	8	0	1
PD13	15	0	1	3	4	6	1
mean (sd)	26 (9)	1 (1)	4 (3)	11 (5)	7 (3)	3 (3)	3 (3)

Table A.10. Overview over the scores of the motor assessment of individuals with PD in DBS-ON condition.

	total	speech	axial	bradykinesia	rigidity	tremor	PIGD
PD01	21	2	6	13	0	0	5
PD02	6	1	2	2	0	1	1
PD03	24	0	4	16	1	2	5
PD04	5	0	0	3	1	0	0
PD05	34	2	8	15	3	6	9
PD06	16	2	5	8	1	0	3
PD07	18	0	3	6	6	2	4
PD08	17	0	1	13	1	2	2
PD09	11	0	2	3	4	1	2
PD10	10	0	0	7	3	0	2
PD11	9	0	3	2	2	2	3
PD12	11	2	3	3	3	0	3
PD13	3	0	0	1	2	0	0
mean (sd)	14 (9)	1 (1)	3 (2)	7 (5)	2 (2)	1 (2)	3 (2)

A.5 Levodopa Equivalent Daily Doses

The following Table A.11 presents the levodopa equivalent daily doses (LEDD) in mg that were calculated according to the tool developed by Tomlinson et al. (2010). Values are given for the total dosages (LEDD total) and the dopamine agonists (LEDD agonists) only for the preoperative and postoperative amount.

Table A.11. The amount in mg of anti-Parkinsonism drugs taken per patient before DBS implantation (preoperative) and after implantation (postoperative) of DBS electrodes.

	preoperative		postoperative	
	LEDD total	LEDD agonists	LEDD total	LEDD agonists
PD01	982	240	475	0
PD02	1099	150	562	149
PD03	1198	0	599	0
PD04	1030	320	40	40
PD05	1224	160	1008	110
PD06	1120	451	450	150
PD07	1452	752	900	150
PD08	540	240	150	0
PD09	1254	215	675	150
PD10	745	270	0	0
PD11	1050	450	901	301
PD12	1105	240	280	180
PD13	420	320	260	160
mean (sd)	1017 (290)	293 (183)	485 (331)	107 (93)

References

Aarsland, D., Påhlhagen, S., Ballard, C. G., Ehrt, U., & Svenningsson, P. (2012). Depression in parkinson disease — epidemiology, mechanisms and management. *Nature Reviews Neurology*, *8*(1), 35–47.

Abbott, R., Petrovitch, H., White, L., Masaki, K., Tanner, C., Curb, J., ... Ross, G. (2001). Frequency of bowel movements and the future risk of parkinson's disease. *Neurology*, *57*(3), 456–462.

Ackermann, H., Hertrich, I., & Hehr, T. (1995). Oral diadochokinesis in neurological dysarthrias. *Folia Phoniatrica et Logopaedica*, *47*(1), 15–23.

Ackermann, H., & Ziegler, W. (1991). Articulatory deficits in parkinsonian dysarthria: An acoustic analysis. *Journal of Neurology, Neurosurgery & Psychiatry*, *54*(12), 1093–1098.

Afifi, A. K. (2003). The basal ganglia: A neural network with more than motor function. *Seminars in Pediatric Neurology*, *10*(1), 3–10.

Ahn, J. S., van Lancker Sidtis, D., & Sidtis, J. J. (2014). Effects of deep brain stimulation on pausing during spontaneous speech in parkinson's disease. *Journal of Medical Speech-Language Pathology*, *21*(3), 179–186.

Albin, A. (2014). PraatR: An architecture for controlling the phonetics software "Praat" with the R programming language. *Journal of the Acoustical Society of America*, *135*(4), 2198.

Alexander, G., & Crutcher, M. (1990). Functional architecture of basal ganglia circuits. *Trends in Neurosciences*, *13*(7), 266–271.

Anand, S., & Stepp, C. E. (2015). Listener perception of monopitch, naturalness, and intelligibility for speakers with parkinson's disease. *Journal of Speech, Language, and Hearing Research*, *58*(4), 1134–1144.

Antolík, T. K., & Fougeron, C. (2013). Consonant distortions in dysarthria due to parkinson's disease, amyotrophic lateral sclerosis and cerebellar ataxia. In *Proceedings of the 14th Annual Conference of the International Speech Communication Association* (pp. 2152–2156).

Åström, M., Tripoliti, E., Hariz, M. I., Zrinzo, L. U., Martinez-Torres, I., Limousin, P., & Wårdell, K. (2010). Patient-specific model-based investigation of speech intelligibility and movement during deep brain stimulation. *Stereotactic and Functional Neurosurgery*, *88*(4), 224–233.

Audacity-Team. (2021). *Audacity®-software (version 3.1.3) [computer application]*. Retrieved from https://audacityteam.org/

Azevedo, L. L. d., Reis, C. A. d. C., Souza, I. S. d., & Cardoso, F. E. C. (2013). Prosody and levodopa in parkinson's disease. *Arquivos de Neuro-Psiquiatria*, *71*(11), 835–840.

Baese-Berk, M., & Goldrick, M. (2009). Mechanisms of interaction in speech production. *Language and Cognitive Processes*, *24*(4), 527–554.

Baghai-Ravary, L., & Beet, S. W. (2012). *Automatic Speech Signal Analysis for Clinical Diagnosis and Assessment of Speech Disorders*. Springer.

Bandini, A., Orlandi, S., Giovannelli, F., Felici, A., Cincotta, M., Clemente, D., ... Manfredi, C. (2016). Markerless analysis of articulatory movements in patients with parkinson's disease. *Journal of Voice*, *30*(6), 766.e1–e11.

Bates, D., Mächler, M., Bolker, B., & Walker, S. (2015). Fitting linear mixed-effects models using lme4. *Journal of Statistical Software*, *67*(1), 1–48.

Baumann, S., Becker, J., Grice, M., & Mücke, D. (2007). Tonal and articulatory marking of focus in german. In *Proceedings of the 16th International Congress of Phonetic Sciences* (pp. 1029–1032).

Baumann, S., & Grice, M. (2006). The intonation of accessibility. *Journal of Pragmatics*, *38*(10), 1636–1657.

Baumann, S., Grice, M., & Steindamm, S. (2006). Prosodic marking of focus domains-categorical or gradient. In *Proceedings of the 3rd International Conference on Speech Prosody* (pp. 301–304).

Baumann, S., & Röhr, C. T. (2015). The perceptual prominence of pitch accent types in german. In *Proceedings of the 18th International Congress of Phonetic Sciences* (pp. 1–5).

Baumann, S., & Winter, B. (2018). What makes a word prominent? Predicting untrained german listeners' perceptual judgments. *Journal of Phonetics*, 70, 20–38.

Bayram, E., Aslanbaba, E., & Akbostanci, M. C. (2019). Levodopa effect on spontaneous speech in parkinson's disease. *Journal of Neurolinguistics*, 51, 194–198.

Beck, A. T., Steer, R. A., Ball, R., & Ranieri, W. F. (1996). Comparison of beck depression inventories-ia and-ii in psychiatric outpatients. *Journal of Personality Assessment*, 67(3), 588–597.

Beckman, M. E., Edwards, J., & Fletcher, J. (1992). Prosodic structure and tempo in a sonority model of articulatory dynamics. In G. J. Docherty & D. R. Ladd (Eds.), *Papers in laboratory phonology II: Gesture, Segment, Prosody* (pp. 68–89). Cambridge University Press.

Belvisi, D., Pellicciari, R., Fabbrini, G., Tinazzi, M., Berardelli, A., & Defazio, G. (2020). Modifiable risk and protective factors in disease development, progression and clinical subtypes of parkinson's disease: What do prospective studies suggest? *Neurobiology of Disease*, 134, 104671.

Benabid, A. L. (2003). Deep brain stimulation for parkinson's disease. *Current Opinion in Neurobiology*, 13(6), 696–706.

Berg, D., Postuma, R. B., Bloem, B., Chan, P., Dubois, B., Gasser, T., ... Deuschl, G. (2014). Time to redefine PD? Introductory statement of the MDS Task Force on the definition of Parkinson's disease. *Movement Disorders*, 29(4), 454–462.

Boersma, P., & Weenink, D. (2022). Praat: Doing phonetics by computer [Computer software manual]. Retrieved from http://www.praat.org/

Braak, H., Bohl, J. R., Müller, C. M., Rüb, U., de Vos, R., & del Tredici, K. (2005). The staging procedure for the inclusion body pathology associated with sporadic parkinson's disease reconsidered. *Movement Disorders*, 221(12), 2042–2051.

Braak, H., Del Tredici, K., Bratzke, H., Hamm-Clement, J., Sandmann-Keil, D., & Rüb, U. (2002). Staging of the intracerebral inclusion body pathology associated with idiopathic parkinson's disease (preclinical and clinical stages). *Journal of Neurology, 249*(3), iii1–iii5.

Braak, H., Del Tredici, K., Rüb, U., De Vos, R., Steur, E. N. J., & Braak, E. (2003). Staging of brain pathology related to sporadic parkinson's disease. *Neurobiology of Aging, 24*(2), 197–211.

Braak, H., Ghebremedhin, E., Rüb, U., Bratzke, H., & Del Tredici, K. (2004). Stages in the development of parkinson's disease-related pathology. *Cell and Tissue Research, 318*(1), 121–134.

Braun, B., & Ladd, D. R. (2003). Prosodic correlates of contrastive and non-contrastive themes in german. In *Proceedings of the 8th European Conference on Speech Communication and Technology* (pp. 789–792).

Brendel, B., Lowit, A., & Howell, P. (2004). The effects of delayed and frequency shifted feedback on speakers with Parkinson's disease. *Journal of Medical Speech-Language Pathology, 12*, 131–138.

Browman, C. P., & Goldstein, L. (1988). Some notes on syllable structure in articulatory phonology. *Phonetica, 45*(2-4), 140–155.

Browman, C. P., & Goldstein, L. (1989). Articulatory gestures as phonological units. *Phonology, 6*(2), 201–251.

Browman, C. P., & Goldstein, L. (1990). Tiers in articulatory phonology, with some implications for casual speech. In J. Kingston & M. E. Beckman (Eds.), *Papers in laboratory phonology I: Between the grammar and physics of speech* (pp. 341–376). Cambridge University Press.

Browman, C. P., & Goldstein, L. (1992). Articulatory phonology: An overview. *Phonetica, 49*(3-4), 155–180.

Brown, P., Oliviero, A., Mazzone, P., Insola, A., Tonali, P., & Di Lazzaro, V. (2001). Dopamine dependency of oscillations between subthalamic nucleus and pallidum in parkinson's disease. *Journal of Neuroscience, 21*(3), 1033–1038.

Brunner, J., Hoole, P., Perrier, P., & Fuchs, S. (2006). Temporal development of compensation strategies for perturbed palate shape in german/sch/-production. In *Proceedings of the 7th International Seminar on Speech Production* (pp. 247–254).

Burke, R. E., Dauer, W. T., & Vonsattel, J. P. G. (2008). A critical evaluation of the braak staging scheme for parkinson's disease. *Annals of Neurology*, *64*(5), 485–491.

Castrioto, A., Volkmann, J., & Krack, P. (2013). Postoperative management of deep brain stimulation in parkinson's disease. In A. M. Lozano & M. Hallett (Eds.), *Handbook of Clinical Neurology* (pp. 129–146). Elsevier.

Cavallieri, F., Budriesi, C., Gessani, A., Contardi, S., Fioravanti, V., Menozzi, E., ... Antonelli, F. (2021). Dopaminergic treatment effects on dysarthric speech: acoustic analysis in a cohort of patients with advanced parkinson's disease. *Frontiers in Neurology*, *11*, 1954.

Cersosimo, M. G., Raina, G. B., Benarroch, E. E., Piedimonte, F., Alemán, G. G., & Micheli, F. E. (2009). Micro lesion effect of the globus pallidus internus and outcome with deep brain stimulation in patients with parkinson disease and dystonia. *Movement Disorders*, *24*(10), 1488–1493.

Chakravarthy, V. S., Joseph, D., & Bapi, R. S. (2010). What do the basal ganglia do? A modeling perspective. *Biological Cybernetics*, *103*(3), 237–253.

Charles, P., Van Blercom, N., Krack, P., Lee, S., Xie, J., Besson, G., ... Pollak, P. (2002). Predictors of effective bilateral subthalamic nucleus stimulation for pd. *Neurology*, *59*(6), 932–934.

Cheang, H. S., & Pell, M. D. (2007). An acoustic investigation of parkinsonian speech in linguistic and emotional contexts. *Journal of Neurolinguistics*, *20*(3), 221–241.

Cho, T. (2005). Prosodic strengthening and featural enhancement: Evidence from acoustic and articulatory realizations of /a, i/ in english. *The Journal of the Acoustical Society of America*, *117*(6), 3867–3878.

Cho, T. (2006). Manifestation of prosodic structure in articulatory variation: Evidence from lip kinematics in english. In L. Goldstein, D. Whalen, & C. T. Best (Eds.), *Laboratory phonology 8* (pp. 519–548). De Gruyter Mouton.

Cho, T., & McQueen, J. M. (2005). Prosodic influences on consonant production in dutch: Effects of prosodic boundaries, phrasal accent and lexical stress. *Journal of Phonetics*, *33*(2), 121–157.

Chu, S. Y., Barlow, S. M., & Lee, J. (2015). Face-referenced measurement of perioral stiffness and speech kinematics in parkinson's disease. *Journal of Speech, Language, and Hearing Research*, *58*(2), 201–212.

Commissioning Board, N. (2013). Clinical commissioning policy: Deep brain stimulation (dbs) in movement disorders (parkinson's disease, tremor and dystonia). *Adult Neurosurgery CRG*.

Connor, N. P., Abbs, J. H., Cole, K. J., & Gracco, V. L. (1989). Parkinsonian deficits in serial multiarticulate movements for speech. *Brain*, *112*(4), 997–1009.

Cote-Reschny, K. J., & Hodge, M. M. (2010). Listener effort and response time when transcribing words spoken by children with dysarthria. *Journal of Medical Speech-Language Pathology*, *18*(4), 24–35.

Dafsari, H. S., dos Santos Ghilardi, M. G., Visser-Vandewalle, V., Rizos, A., Ashkan, K., Silverdale, M., … Timmermann, L. (2020). Beneficial nonmotor effects of subthalamic and pallidal neurostimulation in parkinson's disease. *Brain Stimulation*, *13*(6), 1697–1705.

D'Alatri, L., Paludetti, G., Contarino, M. F., Galla, S., Marchese, M. R., & Bentivoglio, A. R. (2008). Effects of bilateral subthalamic nucleus stimulation and medication on parkinsonian speech impairment. *Journal of Voice*, *22*(3), 365–372.

Darley, F. L., Aronson, A. E., & Brown, J. R. (1969). Differential diagnostic patterns of dysarthria. *Journal of Speech and Hearing Research*, *12*(2), 246–269.

Darley, F. L., Aronson, A. E., & Brown, J. R. (1975). *Motor Speech Disorders*. WB Saunders Company.

Darling, M., & Huber, J. E. (2011). Changes to articulatory kinematics in response to loudness cues in individuals with parkinson's disease. *Journal of Speech, Language, and Hearing Research*, *54*(5), 1247–1259.

De Jong, K. (1995). The supraglottal articulation of prominence in english: Linguistic stress as localized hyperarticulation. *The Journal of the Acoustical Society of America*, *97*(1), 491–504.

De Jong, K., Beckman, M., & Edwards, J. (1993). The interplay between prosodic structure and coarticulation. *Language and Speech*, *36*(2-3), 197–212.

de Keyser, K., Santens, P., Bockstael, A., Botteldooren, D., Talsma, D., De Vos, S., ... De Letter, M. (2016). The relationship between speech production and speech perception deficits in parkinson's disease. *Journal of Speech, Language, and Hearing Research*, *59*(5), 915–931.

de la Fuente-Fernández, R. (2012). Role of DaTSCan and clinical diagnosis in parkinson disease. *Neurology*, *78*(10), 696–701.

de la Fuente-Fernández, R., Schulzer, M., & Stoessl, A. J. (2004). Placebo mechanisms and reward circuitry: Clues from parkinson's disease. *Biological Psychiatry*, *56*(2), 67–71.

De Lau, L. M., & Breteler, M. M. (2006). Epidemiology of parkinson's disease. *The Lancet Neurology*, *5*(6), 525–535.

De Letter, M., Santens, P., De Bodt, M., Boon, P., & Van Borsel, J. (2006). Levodopa-induced alterations in speech rate in advanced parkinson's disease. *Acta Neurologica Belgica*, *106*(1), 19.

De Letter, M., Van Borsel, J., Boon, P., De Bodt, M., Dhooge, I., & Santens, P. (2010). Sequential changes in motor speech across a levodopa cycle in advanced parkinson's disease. *International Journal of Speech-Language Pathology*, *12*(5), 405–413.

Delvaux, V., Huet, K., Piccaluga, M., Van Malderen, S., & Harmegnies, B. (2018). Towards a better characterization of parkinsonian speech: A multidimensional acoustic study. In *Proceedings of 19th Annual Conference of the International Speech Communication Association* (pp. 362–366).

De Rijk, M. d., Launer, L., Berger, K., Breteler, M., Dartigues, J., Baldereschi, M., ... Hofman, A. (2000). Prevalence of parkinson's disease in europe: A collaborative study of population-based cohorts. neurologic diseases in the elderly research group. *Neurology*, *54*(11 Suppl 5), S21–3.

Deuschl, G., Oertel, W., & Reichmann, H. (2016). *Leitlinien für Diagnostik und Therapie in der Neurologie: Idiopathisches*

Parkinson-Syndrom Entwicklungsstufe: S3 Kurzversion. Deutsche Gesellschaft für Neurologie.

Dorsey, E., Constantinescu, R., Thompson, J., Biglan, K., Holloway, R., Kieburtz, K., ... Tanner, C. (2007). Projected number of people with parkinson disease in the most populous nations, 2005 through 2030. *Neurology, 68*(5), 384–386.

Dromey, C. (2000). Articulatory kinematics in patients with parkinson disease using different speech treatment approaches. *Journal of Medical Speech Language Pathology, 8*(3), 155–162.

Dromey, C., & Adams, S. (2000). Loudness perception and hypophonia in parkinson disease. *Journal of Medical Speech-Language Pathology, 8*(4), 255–259.

Dromey, C., & Bjarnason, S. (2011). A preliminary report on disordered speech with deep brain stimulation in individuals with parkinson's disease. *Parkinson's Disease*, 796205.

Duffy, J. R. (2019). *Motor Speech Disorders: Substrates, Differential Diagnosis, and Management*. Elsevier.

Eggers, C., Kahraman, D., Fink, G. R., Schmidt, M., & Timmermann, L. (2011). Akinetic-rigid and tremor-dominant Parkinson's disease patients show different patterns of FP-CIT single photon emission computed tomography. *Movement Disorders, 26*(3), 416–423.

Ehlen, F., Al-Fatly, B., Kühn, A. A., & Klostermann, F. (2020). Impact of deep brain stimulation of the subthalamic nucleus on natural language in patients with parkinson's disease. *PLOS ONE, 15*(12), e0244148.

Eklund, E., Qvist, J., Sandström, L., Viklund, F., Van Doorn, J., & Karlsson, F. (2015). Perceived articulatory precision in patients with parkinson's disease after deep brain stimulation of subthalamic nucleus and caudal zona incerta. *Clinical Linguistics & Phonetics, 29*(2), 150–166.

Elfmarková, N., Gajdoš, M., Mračková, M., Mekyska, J., Mikl, M., & Rektorová, I. (2016). Impact of parkinson's disease and levodopa on resting state functional connectivity related to speech prosody control. *Parkinsonism & Related Disorders, 22*, S52–S55.

Fabbri, M., Guimarães, I., Cardoso, R., Coelho, M., Guedes, L. C., Rosa, M. M., ... Ferreira, J. J. (2017). Speech and voice response to a levodopa challenge in late-stage parkinson's disease. *Frontiers in Neurology, 8,* 432.

Fahn, S. (2003). Description of parkinson's disease as a clinical syndrome. *Annals of the New York Academy of Sciences, 991*(1), 1–14.

Fahn, S., Elton, R., & Committee, U. D. (1987). Unified parkinson's disease rating scale. In S. Fahn, C. Marsden, D. Calne, & M. Goldstein (Eds.), *Recent developments in Parkinson's disease* (Vol. 2, pp. 153–163). Florham Park.

Fenoy, A. J., McHenry, M. A., & Schiess, M. C. (2016). Speech changes induced by deep brain stimulation of the subthalamic nucleus in parkinson disease: Involvement of the dentatorubrothalamic tract. *Journal of Neurosurgery, 126*(6), 2017–2027.

Ferreira, F., & Swets, B. (2002). How incremental is language production? Evidence from the production of utterances requiring the computation of arithmetic sums. *Journal of Memory and Language, 46*(1), 57–84.

Fivela, B. G., Iraci, M., Sallustio, V., Grimaldi, M., Zmarich, C., & Patrocinio, D. (2014). Italian vowel and consonant (co)articulation in parkinson's disease: Extreme or reduced articulatory variability? In *Proceedings of the 10th International Seminar on Speech Production* (pp. 146–149).

Fivela, B. G., Sallustio, V., Pede, S., & Patrocinio, D. (2021). Phonetic complexity, speech accuracy and intelligibility assessment of italian dysarthric speech. In *Proceedings of the 22nd Annual Conference of the International Speech Communication Association* (pp. 2926–2930).

Fletcher, A. R., McAuliffe, M. J., Lansford, K. L., & Liss, J. M. (2015). The relationship between speech segment duration and vowel centralization in a group of older speakers. *The Journal of the Acoustical Society of America, 138*(4), 2132–2139.

Folk, L., & Schiel, F. (2011). The lombard effect in spontaneous dialog speech. In *Proceedings of the 12th Annual Conference of the International Speech Communication Association* (pp. 2701–2704).

Follett, K. A., Weaver, F. M., Stern, M., Hur, K., Harris, C. L., Luo, P., ... Reda, D. J. (2010). Pallidal versus subthalamic deep-brain stimulation for parkinson's disease. *New England Journal of Medicine, 362*(22), 2077–2091.

Folstein, M. F., Folstein, S. E., & McHugh, P. R. (1975). 'Mini-mental state': A practical method for grading the cognitive state of patients for the clinician. *Journal of Psychiatric Research, 12*(3), 189–198.

Forrest, K., & Weismer, G. (1995). Dynamic aspects of lower lip movement in parkinsonian and neurologically normal geriatric speakers' production of stress. *Journal of Speech, Language, and Hearing Research, 38*(2), 260–272.

Forrest, K., Weismer, G., & Turner, G. S. (1989). Kinematic, acoustic, and perceptual analyses of connected speech produced by parkinsonian and normal geriatric adults. *The Journal of the Acoustical Society of America, 85*(6), 2608–2622.

Fougeron, C., & Keating, P. A. (1997). Articulatory strengthening at edges of prosodic domains. *The Journal of the Acoustical Society of America, 101*(6), 3728–3740.

Fowler, C. A. (1995). Acoustic and kinematic correlates of contrastive stress accent in spoken english. In F. Bell-Berti & R. J. Lawrence (Eds.), *Producing Speech: Contemporary Issues: For Katherine Safford Harris* (pp. 355–373). AIP Press: New York.

Fox, C., Ebersbach, G., Ramig, L., & Sapir, S. (2012). LSVT LOUD and LSVT BIG: Behavioral treatment programs for speech and body movement in parkinson disease. *Parkinson's Disease, 391946*.

Frenklach, A., Louie, S., Koop, M. M., & Bronte-Stewart, H. (2009). Excessive postural sway and the risk of falls at different stages of parkinson's disease. *Movement Disorders, 24*(3), 377–385.

Frey, J., Cagle, J., Johnson, K. A., Wong, J. K., Hilliard, J. D., Butson, C. R., ... de Hemptinne, C. (2022). Past, present, and future of deep brain stimulation: hardware, software, imaging, physiology and novel approaches. *Frontiers in Neurology, 13*, 825178.

Frota, S., Cruz, M., Cardoso, R., Guimarães, I., Ferreira, J. J., Pinto, S., & Vigário, M. (2021). (Dys)prosody in parkinson's disease: Effects of medication and disease duration on intonation and prosodic phrasing. *Brain Sciences, 11*(8), 1100.

Gaviria, A. M. (2015). *Acoustic realization of contrastive stress in individuals with parkinson's disease* (Master's thesis). Louisiana State University, Communication Sciences and Disorders.

Gayed, I., Joseph, U., Fanous, M., Wan, D., Schiess, M., Ondo, W., & Won, K.-S. (2015). The impact of DaTscan in the diagnosis of parkinson disease. *Clinical Nuclear Medicine, 40*(5), 390–393.

Gentil, M., Garcia-Ruiz, P., Pollak, P., & Benabid, A.-L. (1999). Effect of stimulation of the subthalamic nucleus on oral control of patients with parkinsonism. *Journal of Neurology, Neurosurgery & Psychiatry, 67*(3), 329–333.

Gentil, M., Pinto, S., Pollak, P., & Benabid, A.-L. (2003). Effect of bilateral stimulation of the subthalamic nucleus on parkinsonian dysarthria. *Brain and Language, 85*(2), 190–196.

Gerfen, C. R., & Wilson, C. J. (1996). The basal ganglia. In L. Swanson, A. Björklund, & T. Hökfelt (Eds.), *Handbook of Chemical Neuroanatomy* (Vol. 12, pp. 371–468). Elsevier.

Gibb, W., & Lees, A. (1988). A comparison of clinical and pathological features of young-and old-onset parkinson's disease. *Neurology, 38*(9), 1402–1402.

Goberman, A., & Blomgren, M. (2003). Parkinsonian speech disfluencies: Effects of L-dopa-related fluctuations. *Journal of Fluency Disorders, 28*(1), 55–70.

Goberman, A., Coelho, C., & Robb, M. (2002). Phonatory characteristics of parkinsonian speech before and after morning medication: The ON and OFF states. *Journal of Communication Disorders, 35*(3), 217–239.

Goberman, A., Coelho, C., & Robb, M. (2005). Prosodic characteristics of parkinsonian speech: The effect of levodopa-based medication. *Journal of Medical Speech-Language Pathology, 13*(1), 51–69.

Goetz, C. G., Fahn, S., Martinez-Martin, P., Poewe, W., Sampaio, C., Stebbins, G. T., ... LaPelle, N. (2007). Movement disorder society-sponsored revision of the unified parkinson's disease rating scale (MDS-UPDRS): Process, format, and clinimetric testing plan. *Movement Disorders, 22*(1), 41–47.

Goetz, C. G., Poewe, W., Rascol, O., Sampaio, C., Stebbins, G. T., Counsell, C., ... Seidl, L. (2004). Movement Disorder Society Task Force report on the Hoehn and Yahr staging scale: Status and Recommendations the Movement Disorder Society Task Force on Rating Scales for Parkinson's disease. *Movement Disorders, 19*(9), 1020–1028.

Goetz, C. G., Tilley, B. C., Shaftman, S. R., Stebbins, G. T., Fahn, S., Martinez-Martin, P., ... LaPelle, N. (2008). Movement disorder society-sponsored revision of the unified parkinson's disease rating scale (MDS-UPDRS): Scale presentation and clinimetric testing results. *Movement Disorders, 23*(15), 2129–2170.

Goldstein, L., & Fowler, C. A. (2003). Articulatory phonology: A phonology for public language use. In N. O. Schiller & A. S. Meyer (Eds.), *Phonetics and Phonology in Language Comprehension and Production: Differences and Similarities* (pp. 159–207). De Gruyter Mouton.

Goldstein, L., Nam, H., Saltzman, E., & Chitoran, I. (2009). Coupled oscillator planning model of speech timing and syllable structure. *Frontiers in Phonetics and Speech Science*, 239–249.

Gracco, V. L., & Abbs, J. H. (1988). Central patterning of speech movements. *Experimental Brain Research, 71*(3), 515–526.

Groenewegen, H. J. (2003). The basal ganglia and motor control. *Neural Plasticity, 10*(1-2), 107–120.

Guehl, D., Cuny, E., Benazzouz, A., Rougier, A., Tison, F., Machado, S., ... Burbaud, P. (2006). Side-effects of subthalamic stimulation in parkinson's disease: clinical evolution and predictive factors. *European Journal of Neurology, 13*(9), 963–971.

Gussenhoven, C. (2004). *The Phonology of Tone and Intonation*. Cambridge University Press.

Haehner, A., Hummel, T., Hummel, C., Sommer, U., Junghanns, S., & Reichmann, H. (2007). Olfactory loss may be a first sign of idiopathic parkinson's disease. *Movement Disorders, 22*(6), 839–842.

Hall, N. (2010). Articulatory phonology. *Language and Linguistics Compass, 4*(9), 818–830.

Harrington, J., & Cassidy, S. (1999). The acoustic theory of speech production. In J. Harrington & S. Cassidy (Eds.), *Techniques in Speech*

Acoustics. Text, Speech and Language Technology (Vol. 8, pp. 29–56). Springer.

Harrington, J., Fletcher, J., & Beckman, M. (2000). Manner and place conflicts in the articulation of accent in australian english. In M. B. Broe & J. B. Pierrehumbert (Eds.), *Papers in laboratory phonology V: Acquisition and the Lexicon* (pp. 40–51). Cambridge University Press.

Hartinger, M., Tripoliti, E., Hardcastle, W. J., & Limousin, P. (2011). Effects of medication and subthalamic nucleus deep brain stimulation on tongue movements in speakers with parkinson's disease using electropalatography: A pilot study. *Clinical Linguistics & Phonetics, 25*(3), 210–230.

Hasbi, A., O'Dowd, B. F., & George, S. R. (2011). Dopamine D1-D2 receptor heteromer signaling pathway in the brain: Emerging physiological relevance. *Molecular Brain, 4*(1), 1–6.

Hely, M. A., Morris, J. G., Reid, W. G., & Trafficante, R. (2005). Sydney multicenter study of parkinson's disease: Non-L-dopa–responsive problems dominate at 15 years. *Movement Disorders, 20*(2), 190–199.

Hely, M. A., Reid, W. G., Adena, M. A., Halliday, G. M., & Morris, J. G. (2008). The sydney multicenter study of parkinson's disease: The inevitability of dementia at 20 years. *Movement Disorders, 23*(6), 837–844.

Henriques, R. N., & van Lieshout, P. (2013). A comparison of methods for decoupling tongue and lower lip from jaw movements in 3d articulography. *Journal of Speech, Language, and Hearing Research, 56*(5), 1503–1516.

Hermes, A., Becker, J., Mücke, D., Baumann, S., & Grice, M. (2008). Articulatory gestures and focus marking in german. In *Proceedings of the 4th conference on speech prosody* (pp. 457–460).

Hermes, A., Mertens, J., & Mücke, D. (2018). Age-related effects on sensorimotor control of speech production. In *Proceedings of the 19th Annual Conference of the International Speech Communication Association* (pp. 1526–1530).

Hermes, A., Mücke, D., & Auris, B. (2017). The variabilityof syllable patterns in tashlhiyt berber and polish. *Journal of Phonetics, 64*, 127–144.

Hermes, A., Mücke, D., & Grice, M. (2013). Gestural coordination of italian word-initial clusters: The case of 'impure s'. *Phonology, 30*(1), 1–25.

Hermes, A., Mücke, D., Thies, T., & Barbe, M. T. (2019). Coordination patterns in essential tremor patients with deep brain stimulation: Syllables with low and high complexity. *Laboratory Phonology, 10*(1).

Hertrich, I., & Ackermann, H. (1993). Acoustic analysis of speech prosody in huntington's and parkinson's disease: A preliminary report. *Clinical Linguistics & Phonetics, 7*(4), 285–297.

Hertrich, I., & Ackermann, H. (2017). Dysarthrie des Parkinson-Syndroms — Klinische Befunde, instrumentelle Daten. In A. Nebel & G. Deuschl (Eds.), *Dysarthrie und Dysphagie bei Morbus Parkinson* (Vol. 2, pp. 56–75). Georg Thieme Verlag.

Hertrich, I., Ackermann, H., & Ziegler, W. (2021). Dysarthria. In J. S. Damico, N. Müller, & M. J. Ball (Eds.), *The Handbook of Language and Speech Disorders* (pp. 334–367). Wiley Online Library.

Hirsch, M. E., Thompson, A., Kim, Y., & Lansford, K. L. (2022). The reliability and validity of speech-language pathologists' estimations of intelligibility in dysarthria. *Brain Sciences, 12*(8), 1011.

Hlavnicka, J. (2018). *Automated analysis of speech disroders in neurodegenerative diseases* (dissertation). Czech Technical University in Pargue, Faculty of Electrical Engineering, Department of Circuit Theory.

Ho, A. K., Bradshaw, J. L., & Iansek, R. (2008). For better or worse: The effect of levodopa on speech in parkinson's disease. *Movement Disorders, 23*(4), 574–580.

Ho, A. K., Iansek, R., Marigliani, C., Bradshaw, J. L., & Gates, S. (1998). Speech impairment in a large sample of patients with parkinson's disease. *Behavioural Neurology, 11*(3), 131–137.

Hoehn, M. (1992). The natural history of parkinson's disease in the pre-levodopa and post-levodopa eras. *Neurologic Clinics, 10*(2), 331–339.

Hoole, P., & Bombien, L. (2017). A cross-language study of laryngeal-oral coordination across varying prosodic and syllable-structure conditions. *Journal of Speech, Language, and Hearing Research, 6*(3), 525–539.

Hsu, S.-C., Jiao, Y., McAuliffe, M. J., Berisha, V., Wu, R.-M., & Levy, E. S. (2017). Acoustic and perceptual speech characteristics of native mandarin speakers with parkinson's disease. *The Journal of the Acoustical Society of America*, *141*(3), EL293–EL299.

Hughes, A. J., Daniel, S. E., Kilford, L., & Lees, A. J. (1992). Accuracy of clinical diagnosis of idiopathic parkinson's disease: A clinicopathological study of 100 cases. *Journal of Neurology, Neurosurgery & Psychiatry*, *55*(3), 181–184.

Im, H., Adams, S., Abeyesekera, A., Pieterman, M., Gilmore, G., & Jog, M. (2019). Effect of levodopa on speech dysfluency in parkinson's disease. *Movement Disorders Clinical Practice*, *6*(2), 150–154.

Iorio-Morin, C., Fomenko, A., & Kalia, S. K. (2020). Deep-brain stimulation for essential tremor and other tremor syndromes: A narrative review of current targets and clinical outcomes. *Brain Sciences*, *10*(12), 925.

Iskarous, K. (2017). The relation between the continuous and the discrete: A note on the first principles of speech dynamics. *Journal of Phonetics*, *64*, 8–20.

Jankovic, J., McDermott, M., Carter, J., Gauthier, S., Goetz, C., Golbe, L., ... Weiner, W. (1990). Variable expression of parkinson's disease: A base-line analysis of the dat atop cohort. *Neurology*, *40*(10), 1529–1529.

Janković, M., Svetel, M., & Kostić, V. (2015). Frequency of rem sleep behavior disorders in patients with parkinson's disease. *Vojnosanitetski Pregled*, *72*(5), 442–446.

Jorge, A., Dastolfo-Hromack, C., Lipski, W. J., Kratter, I. H., Smith, L. J., Gartner-Schmidt, J. L., & Richardson, R. M. (2020). Anterior sensorimotor subthalamic nucleus stimulation is associated with improved voice function. *Neurosurgery*, *87*(4), 788–795.

Kalbe, E., Calabrese, P., Kohn, N., Hilker, R., Riedel, O., Wittchen, H.-U., ... Kessler, J. (2008). Screening for cognitive deficits in parkinson's disease with the parkinson neuropsychometric dementia assessment (PANDA) instrument. *Parkinsonism & Related Disorders*, *14*(2), 93–101.

Kalia, L., & Lang, A. (2015). Parkinson's disease. *The Lancet*, *386*(9996), 896–912.

Karlsson, F., & Hartelius, L. (2019). How well does diadochokinetic task performance predict articulatory imprecision? Differentiating individuals with parkinson's disease from control subjects. *Folia Phoniatrica et Logopaedica*, *71*(5-6), 251–260.

Karlsson, F., Olofsson, K., Blomstedt, P., Linder, J., Nordh, E., & van Doorn, J. (2014). Articulatory closure proficiency in patients with parkinson's disease following deep brain stimulation of the subthalamic nucleus and caudal zona incerta. *Journal of Speech, Language, and Hearing Research*, *57*(4), 1178–1190.

Karlsson, F., Unger, E., Wahlgren, S., Blomstedt, P., Linder, J., Nordh, E., ... van Doorn, J. (2011). Deep brain stimulation of caudal zona incerta and subthalamic nucleus in patients with parkinson's disease: effects on diadochokinetic rate. *Parkinson's Disease*, 605607.

Katsika, A. (2018). The kinematic profile of prominence in greek. In *Proceedings of 9th International Conference on Speech Prosody* (pp. 764–768).

Katzenschlager, R., & Lees, A. J. (2002). Treatment of parkinson's disease: Levodopa as the first choice. *Journal of Neurology*, *249*(2), ii19–ii24.

Kearney, E., Giles, R., Haworth, B., Faloutsos, P., Baljko, M., & Yunusova, Y. (2017). Sentence-level movements in parkinson's disease: Loud, clear, and slow speech. *Journal of Speech, Language, and Hearing Research*, *60*(12), 3426–3440.

Keitel, A., Wojtecki, L., Hirschmann, J., Hartmann, C. J., Ferrea, S., Südmeyer, M., & Schnitzler, A. (2013). Motor and cognitive placebo-/nocebo-responses in parkinson's disease patients with deep brain stimulation. *Behavioural Brain Research*, *250*, 199–205.

Kempler, D., & van Lancker, D. (2002). Effect of speech task on intelligibility in dysarthria: A case study of parkinson's disease. *Brain and Language*, *80*(3), 449–464.

Kent, R. D., Kent, J. F., Weismer, G., & Duffy, J. R. (2000). What dysarthrias can tell us about the neural control of speech. *Journal of Phonetics*, *28*(3), 273–302.

Kent, R. D., & Kim, Y.-J. (2003). Toward an acoustic typology of motor speech disorders. *Clinical Linguistics & Phonetics, 17*(6), 427–445.

Kent, R. D., Weismer, G., Kent, J. F., Vorperian, H. K., & Duffy, J. R. (1999). Acoustic studies of dysarthric speech: Methods, progress, and potential. *Journal of Communication Disorders, 32*(3), 141–186.

Kern, D. S., & Kumar, R. (2007). Deep brain stimulation. *The Neurologist, 13*(5), 237–252.

Kim, D., Kuruvilla-Dugdale, M., de Riesthal, M., Jones, R., Bagnato, F., & Mefferd, A. (2021). Articulatory correlates of stress pattern disturbances in talkers with dysarthria. *Journal of Speech, Language, and Hearing Research, 64*(6S), 2287–2300.

Kim, Y., Kent, R. D., & Weismer, G. (2011). An acoustic study of the relationships among neurologic disease, dysarthria type, and severity of dysarthria. *Journal of Speech, Language, and Hearing Research*, 417–429.

Kim, Y., Weismer, G., Kent, R. D., & Duffy, J. R. (2009). Statistical models of F2 slope in relation to severity of dysarthria. *Folia Phoniatrica et Logopaedica, 61*(6), 329–335.

Klopfenstein, M. (2015). Relationship between acoustic measures and speech naturalness ratings in parkinson's disease: A within-speaker approach. *Clinical Linguistics & Phonetics, 29*(12), 938–954.

Klopfenstein, M. (2016). Speech naturalness ratings and perceptual correlates of highly natural and unnatural speech in hypokinetic dysarthria secondary to parkinson's disease. *Journal of Interactional Research in Communication Disorders, 7*(1), 123.

Klopfenstein, M., Bernard, K., & Heyman, C. (2020). The study of speech naturalness in communication disorders: A systematic review of the literature. *Clinical Linguistics & Phonetics, 34*(4), 327–338.

Knowles, T., Adams, S., Abeyesekera, A., Mancinelli, C., Gilmore, G., & Jog, M. (2018). Deep brain stimulation of the subthalamic nucleus parameter optimization for vowel acoustics and speech intelligibility in parkinson's disease. *Journal of Speech, Language, and Hearing Research, 61*(3), 510–524.

Kochanski, G., Grabe, E., Coleman, J., & Rosner, B. (2005). Loudness predicts prominence: Fundamental frequency lends little. *The Journal of the Acoustical Society of America*, 118(2), 1038–1054.

Kohler, K. J. (1991). Terminal intonation patterns in single-accent utterances of german: Phonetics, phonology and semantics. *Arbeitsberichte des Instituts für Phonetik und digitale Sprachverarbeitung der Universität Kiel (AIPUK)*, 25(1), 15–185.

Kornatz, K. W., Poston, B., & Stelmach, G. E. (2021). Age and not the preferred limb influences the kinematic structure of pointing movements. *Journal of Functional Morphology and Kinesiology*, 6(4), 100.

Krack, P., Kumar, R., Ardouin, C., Dowsey, P. L., McVicker, J. M., Benabid, A.-L., & Pollak, P. (2001). Mirthful laughter induced by subthalamic nucleus stimulation. *Movement Disorders*, 16(5), 867–875.

Krack, P., Pollak, P., Limousin, P., Benazzouz, A., & Benabid, A. (1997). Stimulation of subthalamic nucleus alleviates tremor in parkinson's disease. *The Lancet*, 350(9092), 1675.

Krivokapić, J., Tiede, M. K., & Tyrone, M. E. (2017). A kinematic study of prosodic structure in articulatory and manual gestures: Results from a novel method of data collection. *Laboratory Phonology*, 8(1), 1-26.

Kukull, W., Larson, E., Teri, L., Bowen, J., McCormick, W., & Pfanschmidt, M. (1994). The mini-mental state examination score and the clinical diagnosis of dementia. *Journal of Clinical Epidemiology*, 47(9), 1061–1067.

Kumar, R., Lozano, A., Kim, Y., Hutchison, W., Sime, E., Halket, E., & Lang, A. (1998). Double-blind evaluation of subthalamic nucleus deep brain stimulation in advanced parkinson's disease. *Neurology*, 51(3), 850–855.

Kumar, R., Lozano, A., Sime, E., Halket, E., & Lang, A. (1999). Comparative effects of unilateral and bilateral subthalamic nucleus deep brain stimulation. *Neurology*, 53(3), 561–561.

Kwan, L. C., & Whitehill, T. L. (2011). Perception of speech by individuals with parkinson's disease: A review. *Parkinson's Disease*, 389767.

Kügler, F. (2008). The role of duration as a phonetic correlate of focus. In *Proceedings of the 4th International Conference on Speech Prosody* (pp. 591–594).

Kühnert, B., Hoole, P., & Mooshammer, C. (2007). Gestural overlap and c-center in selected french consonant clusters. In *Proceedings of 7th International Seminar on Speech Production* (pp. 327–334).

Ladd, D. R. (2008). *Intonational Phonology*. Cambridge University Press.

Ladefoged, P., & Johnson, K. (2014). *A Course in Phonetics*. Cengage Learning EMEA.

Laganaro, M., Fougeron, C., Pernon, M., Levêque, N., Borel, S., Fournet, M., ... Delvaux, V. (2021). Sensitivity and specificity of an acoustic-and perceptual-based tool for assessing motor speech disorders in french: The monpage-screening protocol. *Clinical Linguistics & Phonetics*, 35(11), 1060–1075.

Lambrecht, K. (1996). *Information Structure and Sentence Form: Topic, Focus, and the Mental Representations of Discourse Referents* (Vol. 71). Cambridge University Press.

Landa, S., Pennington, L., Miller, N., Robson, S., Thompson, V., & Steen, N. (2014). Association between objective measurement of the speech intelligibility of young people with dysarthria and listener ratings of ease of understanding. *International Journal of Speech-Language Pathology*, 16(4), 408–416.

Lange, S. F., Kremer, N. I., van Laar, T., Lange, F., Steendam-Oldekamp, T. E., Oterdoom, D. M., ... Drost, G. (2022). The intraoperative microlesion effect positively correlates with the short-term clinical effect of deep brain stimulation in parkinson's disease. *Neuromodulation: Technology at the Neural Interface*, 1–7.

Lansford, K. L., & Liss, J. M. (2014). Vowel acoustics in dysarthria: Speech disorder diagnosis and classification. *Journal of Speech, Language, and Hearing Research*, 57(1), 57 – 67.

Lawton, M., Ben-Shlomo, Y., May, M. T., Baig, F., Barber, T. R., Klein, J. C., ... Hu, M. T. (2018). Developing and validating parkinson's disease subtypes and their motor and cognitive progression. *Journal of Neurology, Neurosurgery & Psychiatry*, 89(12), 1279–1287.

Leanderson, R., Meyerson, B., & Persson, A. (1971). Effect of l-dopa on speech in parkinsonism: An emg study of labial articulatory function. *Journal of Neurology, Neurosurgery & Psychiatry, 34*(6), 679–681.

Lehner, K., Ziegler, W., & Group, K. S. (2021). Clinical measures of communication limitations in dysarthria assessed through crowdsourcing: Specificity, sensitivity, and retest-reliability. *Clinical Linguistics & Phonetics*, 1–22.

Leiner, D. (2019). *Sosci survey (version 3.3.02) [computer software]*. https://www.soscisurvey.de.

Lenth, R. V. (2022). emmeans: Estimated marginal means, aka least-squares means [Computer software manual]. Retrieved from https://CRAN.R-project.org/package=emmeans (R package version 1.8.3)

Leritz, E., Loftis, C., Crucian, G., Friedman, W., & Bowers, D. (2004). Self-awareness of deficits in Parkinson disease. *The Clinical Neuropsychologist, 18*(3), 352–361.

Levelt, W. J. M. (1993). *Speaking: From Intention to Articulation*. MIT press.

Levelt, W. J. M., & Meyer, A. S. (2000). Word for word: Multiple lexical access in speech production. *European Journal of Cognitive Psychology, 12*(4), 433–452.

Lewis, S., Foltynie, T., Blackwell, A. D., Robbins, T. W., Owen, A. M., & Barker, R. A. (2005). Heterogeneity of parkinson's disease in the early clinical stages using a data driven approach. *Journal of Neurology, Neurosurgery & Psychiatry, 76*(3), 343–348.

Liang, G. S., Chou, K. L., Baltuch, G. H., Jaggi, J. L., Loveland-Jones, C., Leng, L., ... Siderowf, A. D. (2006). Long-term outcomes of bilateral subthalamic nucleus stimulation in patients with advanced parkinson's disease. *Stereotactic and Functional Neurosurgery, 84*(5-6), 221–227.

Limousin, P., & Martinez-Torres, I. (2008). Deep brain stimulation for parkinson's disease. *Neurotherapeutics, 5*(2), 309–319.

Lind, G., Schechtmann, G., Lind, C., Winter, J., Meyerson, B. A., & Linderoth, B. (2008). Subthalamic stimulation for essential tremor. *Stereotactic and Functional Neurosurgery, 86*(4), 253–258.

Lindblom, B. (1990). Explaining phonetic variation: A sketch of the H&H theory. In W. J. Hardcastle & A. Marchal (Eds.), *Speech Production and Speech Modelling* (pp. 403–439). Springer.

Liss, J. M., White, L., Mattys, S. L., Lansford, K., Lotto, A. J., Spitzer, S. M., & Caviness, J. N. (2009). Quantifying speech rhythm abnormalities in the dysarthrias. *Journal of Speech, Language, and Hearing Research*, 52(2), 1334 – 1352.

Löfqvist, A. (2010). Theories and models of speech production. In W. J. Hardcastle, J. Laver, & F. E. Gibbon (Eds.), *The Handbook of Phonetic Sciences* (2nd ed., pp. 353–377). Wiley-Blackwell.

Logemann, J. A., & Fisher, H. B. (1981). Vocal tract control in parkinson's disease. *Journal of Speech and Hearing Disorders*, 46(4), 348–352.

Logemann, J. A., Fisher, H. B., Boshes, B., & Blonsky, E. R. (1978). Frequency and cooccurrence of vocal tract dysfunctions in the speech of a large sample of parkinson patients. *Journal of Speech and Hearing Disorders*, 43(1), 47–57.

Lowit, A., Brendel, B., Dobinson, C., & Howell, P. (2006). An investigation into the influences of age, pathology and cognition on speech production. *Journal of Medical Speech-Language Pathology*, 14, 253.

Lowit, A., Ijitona, T., Kuschmann, A., Corson, S., & Soraghan, J. (2018). What does it take to stress a word? Digital manipulation of stress markers in ataxic dysarthria. *International Journal of Language & Communication Disorders*, 53(4), 875–887.

Lozano, A. M., Lipsman, N., Bergman, H., Brown, P., Chabardes, S., Chang, J. W., ... others (2019). Deep brain stimulation: Current challenges and future directions. *Nature Reviews Neurology*, 15(3), 148–160.

Lundgren, S., Saeys, T., Karlsson, F., Olofsson, K., Blomstedt, P., Linder, J., ... van Doorn, J. (2011). Deep brain stimulation of caudal zona incerta and subthalamic nucleus in patients with parkinson's disease: effects on voice intensity. *Parkinson's Disease*, 658956.

Macchi, M. (1988). Labial articulation patterns associated with segmental features and syllable structure in english. *Phonetica*, 45(2-4), 109-121.

Maier, F., & Prigatano, G. P. (2017). Impaired self-awareness of motor disturbances in Parkinson's disease. *Archives of Clinical Neuropsychology*, *32*(7), 802–809.

Maltête, D., Derrey, S., Chastan, N., Debono, B., Gérardin, E., Fréger, P., ... Hannequin, D. (2008). Microsubthalamotomy: An immediate predictor of long-term subthalamic stimulation efficacy in parkinson disease. *Movement Disorders*, *23*(7), 1047–1050.

Manuguerra, M., Heller, G., & Ma, J. (2020). Continuous ordinal regression for analysis of visual analogue scales: The R package ordinalcont. *Journal of Statistical Software*, *96*, 1–25.

Marin, S., & Pouplier, M. (2010). Temporal organization of complex onsets and codas in american english: Testing the predictions of a gestural coupling model. *Motor Control*, *14*(3), 380–407.

Martel Sauvageau, V., Macoir, J., Langlois, M., Prud'Homme, M., Cantin, L., & Roy, J.-P. (2014). Changes in vowel articulation with subthalamic nucleus deep brain stimulation in dysarthric speakers with parkinson's disease. *Parkinson's Disease*, 487035.

Martel Sauvageau, V., Roy, J.-P., Cantin, L., Prud'Homme, M., Langlois, M., & Macoir, J. (2015). Articulatory changes in vowel production following stn dbs and levodopa intake in parkinson's disease. *Parkinson's Disease*, 382320.

Martel-Sauvageau, V., & Tjaden, K. (2017). Vocalic transitions as markers of speech acoustic changes with stn-dbs in parkinson's disease. *Journal of Communication Disorders*, *70*, 1–11.

Mattingly, I. G. (1981). Phonetic representation and speech synthesis by rule. In T. Myers, J. Laver, & J. Anderson (Eds.), *Advances in Psychology* (Vol. 7, pp. 415–420). Elsevier.

Mattys, S. L., Davis, M. H., Bradlow, A. R., & Scott, S. K. (2012). Speech recognition in adverse conditions: A review. *Language and Cognitive Processes*, *27*(7-8), 953–978.

McGuire, J. T., & Botvinick, M. M. (2010). Prefrontal cortex, cognitive control, and the registration of decision costs. *Proceedings of the National Academy of Sciences*, *107*(17), 7922–7926.

McRae, P. A., Tjaden, K., & Schoonings, B. (2002). Acoustic and perceptual consequences of articulatory rate change in parkinson disease. *Journal of Speech, Language, and Hearing Research*, 45(1), 35 – 50.

Mefferd, A. (2015). Articulatory-to-acoustic relations in talkers with dysarthria: A first analysis. *Journal of Speech, Language, and Hearing Research*, 58(3), 576–589.

Mefferd, A. (2017). Tongue-and jaw-specific contributions to acoustic vowel contrast changes in the diphthong /ai/in response to slow, loud, and clear speech. *Journal of Speech, Language, and Hearing Research*, 60(11), 3144–3158.

Mefferd, A., & Dietrich, M. (2019). Tongue-and jaw-specific articulatory underpinnings of reduced and enhanced acoustic vowel contrast in talkers with parkinson's disease. *Journal of Speech, Language, and Hearing Research*, 62(7), 2118–2132.

Mehanna, R., Moore, S., Hou, J. G., Sarwar, A. I., & Lai, E. C. (2014). Comparing clinical features of young onset, middle onset and late onset parkinson's disease. *Parkinsonism & Related Disorders*, 20(5), 530–534.

Mercado, R., Constantoyannis, C., Mandat, T., Kumar, A., Schulzer, M., Stoessl, A. J., & Honey, C. R. (2006). Expectation and the placebo effect in parkinson's disease patients with subthalamic nucleus deep brain stimulation. *Movement Disorders*, 21(9), 1457–1461.

Mestre, T. A., Lang, A. E., & Okun, M. S. (2016). Factors influencing the outcome of deep brain stimulation: Placebo, nocebo, lessebo, and lesion effects. *Movement Disorders*, 31(3), 290–298.

Morello, A. N. D. C., Beber, B. C., Fagundes, V. C., Cielo, C. A., & Rieder, C. R. (2020). Dysphonia and dysarthria in people with parkinson's disease after subthalamic nucleus deep brain stimulation: effect of frequency modulation. *Journal of Voice*, 34(3), 477–484.

Moro, E., Lozano, A. M., Pollak, P., Agid, Y., Rehncrona, S., Volkmann, J., ... Lang, A. E. (2010). Long-term results of a multicenter study on subthalamic and pallidal stimulation in parkinson's disease. *Movement Disorders*, 25(5), 578–586.

Mücke, D. (2018). *Dynamische Modellierung von Artikulation und prosodischer Struktur: Eine Einführung in die Artikulatorische Phonologie*. Language Science Press.

Mücke, D., Hermes, A., Roettger, T. B., Becker, J., Niemann, H., Dembek, T. A., ... Barbe, M. T. (2018). The effects of thalamic deep brain stimulation on speech dynamics in patients with essential tremor: An articulographic study. *PLOS ONE, 13*(1), e0191359.

Mücke, D., Thies, T., Mertens, J., & Hermes, A. (2021). Age-related effects of prosodic prominence in vowel articulation. In *Proceedings of the 12th International Seminar on Speech Production* (pp. 126–129).

Müller, J., Wenning, G. K., Verny, M., McKee, A., Chaudhuri, K. R., Jellinger, K., ... Litvan, I. (2001). Progression of dysarthria and dysphagia in postmortem-confirmed parkinsonian disorders. *Archives of Neurology, 58*(2), 259–264.

Munhall, K. G., Ostry, D. J., & Avraham, P. (1985). Characteristics of velocity profiles of speech movements. *Journal of Experimental Psychology: Human Perception and Performance, 11*(4), 457–474.

Mücke, D., & Grice, M. (2014). The effect of focus marking on supralaryngeal articulation–is it mediated by accentuation? *Journal of Phonetics, 44*, 47–61.

Mücke, D., & Grice, M. (2016). Segment und Geste in der Lautsprache. In U. Domahs & B. Primus (Eds.), *Handbuch Laut, Gebärde, Buchstabe* (Vol. 1, pp. 3–24). De Gruyter.

Mücke, D., Hermes, A., & Cho, T. (2017). Mechanisms of regulation in speech: Linguistic structure and physical control system. *Journal of Phonetics, 64*, 1–7.

Mücke, D., Mefferd, A., Thies, T., Roessig, S., & Hermes, A. (2022). Analysis and modelling of impaired speech movements: Challenges and future directions. *Stem-, Spraak- en Taalpathologie, 27*(Supplement, augustus 2022), 239–240.

Nelson, N. R., & Wedel, A. (2017). The phonetic specificity of competition: Contrastive hyperarticulation of voice onset time in conversational english. *Journal of Phonetics, 64*, 51–70.

Neppert, J. M. (1999). *Elemente einer akustischen Phonetik* (4th ed.). Buske.

Noffs, G., de Campos Duprat, A., Zarzur, A. P., Cury, R. G., Cataldo, B. O., & Fonoff, E. (2017). Effect of levodopa+ carbidopa on the laryngeal electromyographic pattern in parkinson disease. *Journal of Voice, 31*(3), 383–e19.

Noyce, A. J., Bestwick, J. P., Silveira-Moriyama, L., Hawkes, C. H., Giovannoni, G., Lees, A. J., & Schrag, A. (2012). Meta-analysis of early nonmotor features and risk factors for parkinson disease. *Annals of Neurology, 72*(6), 893–901.

Obeso, J. A., Rodriguez-Oroz, M. C., Stamelou, M., Bhatia, K. P., & Burn, D. J. (2014). The expanding universe of disorders of the basal ganglia. *The Lancet, 384*(9942), 523–531.

Okada, Y., Murata, M., & Toda, T. (2015). Effects of levodopa on vowel articulation in patients with parkinson's disease. *Kobe Journal of Medical Sciences, 61*(5), 144–154.

Onslow, M., Adams, R., & Ingham, R. (1992). Reliability of speech naturalness ratings of stuttered speech during treatment. *Journal of Speech, Language, and Hearing Research, 35*(5), 994–1001.

Ostry, D. J., Cooke, J. D., & Munhall, K. G. (1987). Velocity curves of human arm and speech movements. *Experimental Brain Research, 68*(1), 37–46.

Ostry, D. J., & Munhall, K. G. (1985). Control of rate and duration of speech movements. *Journal of the Acoustical Society of America, 77*(2), 640–648.

Pagel, L., Roessig, S., & Mücke, D. (2020). Modifications of tongue body kinematics as a focus marking strategy in german. In *Proceedings of the 12 International Seminar on Speech Production* (pp. 14–18).

Pahwa, R., Factor, S., Lyons, K., Ondo, W., Gronseth, G., Bronte-Stewart, H., ... Weiner, W. (2006). Practice parameter: Treatment of parkinson disease with motor fluctuations and dyskinesia (an evidence-based review): Report of the quality standards subcommittee of the american academy of neurology. *Neurology, 66*(7), 983–995.

Parkinson Study Group, T. (2004). Levodopa and the progression of parkinson's disease. *New England Journal of Medicine, 351*(24), 2498–2508.

Patri, J.-F., Diard, J., & Perrier, P. (2015). Optimal speech motor control and token-to-token variability: A bayesian modeling approach. *Biological Cybernetics, 109*(6), 611–626.

Pell, M. D., Cheang, H. S., & Leonard, C. L. (2006). The impact of parkinson's disease on vocal-prosodic communication from the perspective of listeners. *Brain and Language, 97*(2), 123–134.

Penner, N. M., Hertrich, I., Ackermann, H., & Friedrich Schumm, H. (2001). Dysprosody in parkinson's disease: An investigation of intonation patterns. *Clinical Linguistics & Phonetics, 15*(7), 551–566.

Perrier, P., & Fuchs, S. (2015). Motor equivalence in speech production. In M. A. Redford (Ed.), *The Handbook of Speech Production* (pp. 223–247). John Wiley & Sons, Inc.

Phokaewvarangkul, O., Boonpang, K., & Bhidayasiri, R. (2019). Subthalamic deep brain stimulation aggravates speech problems in parkinson's disease: Objective and subjective analysis of the influence of stimulation frequency and electrode contact location. *Parkinsonism & Related Disorders, 66*, 110–116.

Pieterman, M., Adams, S., & Jog, M. (2018). Method of levodopa response calculation determines strength of association with clinical factors in parkinson disease. *Frontiers in Neurology, 9*, 260.

Pinto, S., Gentil, M., Fraix, V., Benabid, A.-L., & Pollak, P. (2003). Bilateral subthalamic stimulation effects on oral force control in parkinson's disease. *Journal of Neurology, 250*(2), 179–187.

Pinto, S., Gentil, M., Krack, P., Sauleau, P., Fraix, V., Benabid, A.-L., & Pollak, P. (2005). Changes induced by levodopa and subthalamic nucleus stimulation on parkinsonian speech. *Movement Disorders, 20*(11), 1507–1515.

Pollack, A. E. (2001). Anatomy, physiology, and pharmacology of the basal ganglia. *Neurologic Clinics, 19*(3), 523–534.

Polychronis, S., Niccolini, F., Pagano, G., Yousaf, T., & Politis, M. (2019). Speech difficulties in early de novo patients with parkinson's disease. *Parkinsonism & Related Disorders, 64*, 256–261.

Pötter-Nerger, M., & Volkmann, J. (2013). Deep brain stimulation for gait and postural symptoms in parkinson's disease. *Movement Disorders, 28*(11), 1609–1615.

Prolific. (2014). *Prolific [computer software]*. https://www.prolific.co.

R Core Team. (2022). *R: A language and environment for statistical computing [Computer software manual]*. Vienna, Austria. Retrieved from https://www.R-project.org/

Ramasubbu, R., Lang, S., & Kiss, Z. H. (2018). Dosing of electrical parameters in deep brain stimulation (dbs) for intractable depression: a review of clinical studies. *Frontiers in Psychiatry, 9*, 302.

Ramig, L. O., Sapir, S., Countryman, S., Pawlas, A. A., O'Brien, C., Hoehn, M., & Thompson, L. L. (2001). Intensive voice treatment (LSVT®) for patients with parkinson's disease: A 2 year follow up. *Journal of Neurology, Neurosurgery & Psychiatry, 71*(4), 493–498.

Rascol, O., Payoux, P., Ory, F., Ferreira, J. J., Brefel-Courbon, C., & Montastruc, J.-L. (2003). Limitations of current parkinson's disease therapy. *Annals of Neurology, 53*(S3), 3–15.

Reichmann, H. (2009). Dopamine agonist therapy in advanced parkinson's disease. *Journal of Movement Disorders, 2*(1), 10–13.

Robertson
, L. T., St George, R. J., Carlson-Kuhta, P., Hogarth, P., Burchiel, K. J., & Horak, F. B. (2011). Site of deep brain stimulation and jaw velocity in parkinson disease. *Journal of Neurosurgery, 115*(5), 985–994.

Rodriguez-Oroz, M. C., Obeso, J., Lang, A., Houeto, J.-L., Pollak, P., Rehncrona, S., ... Van Blercom, N. (2005). Bilateral deep brain stimulation in parkinson's disease: a multicentre study with 4 years follow-up. *Brain, 128*(10), 2240–2249.

Roessig, S. (2021). *Categoriality and Continuity in Prosodic Prominence*. Language Science Press.

Roessig, S., & Mücke, D. (2019). Modeling dimensions of prosodic prominence. *Frontiers in Communication*, 4, 44.

Roessig, S., Winter, B., & Mücke, D. (2022). Tracing the phonetic space of prosodic focus marking. *Frontiers in Artificial Intelligence*, 5.

Rosen, K. M., Kent, R. D., & Duffy, J. R. (2005). Task-based profile of vocal intensity decline in parkinson's disease. *Folia Phoniatrica et Logopaedica*, 57(1), 28–37.

Rousseau, B., & Watts, C. R. (2002). Susceptibility of speakers with Parkinson disease to delayed feedback. *Journal of Medical Speech-Language Pathology*, 10(1), 41–50.

Roy, N., Nissen, S. L., Dromey, C., & Sapir, S. (2009). Articulatory changes in muscle tension dysphonia: Evidence of vowel space expansion following manual circumlaryngeal therapy. *Journal of Communication Disorders*, 42(2), 124–135.

Rusz, J., Cmejla, R., Růžička, H., Klempíř, J., Majerová, V., Picmausová, J., ... Růžička, E. (2013). Evaluation of speech impairment in early stages of parkinson's disease: A prospective study with the role of pharmacotherapy. *Journal of Neural Transmission*, 120(2), 319–329.

Rusz, J., Cmejla, R., Růžička, H., & Ruzicka, E. (2011). Quantitative acoustic measurements for characterization of speech and voice disorders in early untreated parkinson's disease. *The Journal of the Acoustical Society of America*, 129(1), 350–367.

Rusz, J., Cmejla, R., Tykalová, T., Růžička, H., Klempir, J., Majerova, V., ... Ruzicka, E. (2013). Imprecise vowel articulation as a potential early marker of parkinson's disease: Effect of speaking task. *The Journal of the Acoustical Society of America*, 134(3), 2171–2181.

Rusz, J., Tykalová, T., Novotnỳ, M., Růžička, E., & Dušek, P. (2021). Distinct patterns of speech disorder in early-onset and late-onset de-novo parkinson's disease. *npj Parkinson's Disease*, 7(1), 1–8.

Rusz, J., Tykalová, T., Novotny, M., Zogala, D., Sonka, K., Ruzicka, E., & Dusek, P. (2021). Defining speech subtypes in de novo parkinson disease: Response to long-term levodopa therapy. *Neurology*, 97(21), e2124–e2135.

Röhr, C. T., Baumann, S., Schumacher, P. B., & Grice, M. (2020). Perceptual prominence of accent types and the role of expectations. In *Proceedings of 10th International Conference on Speech Prosody* (pp. 366–370).

Saltzman, E. (1986). Task dynamic coordination of the speech articulators: A preliminary model. *Experimental Brain Research Series, 15*, 129–144.

Saltzman, E., & Kelso, S. J. (1987). Skilled actions: a task-dynamic approach. *Psychological Review, 94*, 84–106.

Saltzman, E., & Munhall, K. (1989). A dynamical approach to gestural patterning in speech production. *Ecological psychology, 1*(4), 333–382.

Sanabria, J., Ruiz, P. G., Gutierrez, R., Marquez, F., Escobar, P., Gentil, M., & Cenjor, C. (2001). The effect of levodopa on vocal function in parkinson's disease. *Clinical Neuropharmacology, 24*(2), 99–102.

Santens, P., De Letter, M., Van Borsel, J., De Reuck, J., & Caemaert, J. (2003). Lateralized effects of subthalamic nucleus stimulation on different aspects of speech in parkinson's disease. *Brain and Language, 87*(2), 253–258.

Sapir, S., Ramig, L. O., Spielman, J. L., & Fox, C. (2010). Formant centralization ratio: A proposal for a new acoustic measure of dysarthric speech. *Journal of Speech, Language, and Hearing Research, 53*, 114–125.

Sapir, S., Spielman, J., Ramig, L. O., Hinds, S. L., Countryman, S., Fox, C., & Story, B. (2003). Effects of intensive voice treatment (the lee silverman voice treatment [LSVT]) on ataxic dysarthria. *American Journal of Speech-Language Pathology, 12*(4), 387 – 399.

Scarborough, R. (2013). Neighborhood-conditioned patterns in phonetic detail: Relating coarticulation and hyperarticulation. *Journal of Phonetics, 41*(6), 491–508.

Schapira, A. H., Chaudhuri, K., & Jenner, P. (2017). Non-motor features of parkinson disease. *Nature Reviews Neuroscience, 18*(7), 435–450.

Schrag, A., & Schott, J. M. (2006). Epidemiological, clinical, and genetic characteristics of early-onset parkinsonism. *The Lancet Neurology, 5*(4), 355–363.

Schreen, J., Thies, T., Hermes, A., & Mücke, D. (2022). Age-related changes on tongue body movements. In *Abstracts of the 8th International Conference on Speech Motor Control* (Vol. 22, pp. 247–248).

Schüpbach, W., Maltête, D., Houeto, J., du Montcel, S. T., Mallet, L., Welter, M., ... Agid, Y. (2007). Neurosurgery at an earlier stage of parkinson disease: A randomized, controlled trial. *Neurology, 68*(4), 267–271.

Schwab, R. S. (1969). Projection technique for evaluating surgery in parkinson's disease. In *Proceedings of the 3rd Symposium on Parkinson's Disease* (pp. 152–157).

Selikhova, M., Williams, D. R., Kempster, P. A., Holton, J. L., Revesz, T., & Lees, A. J. (2009). A clinico-pathological study of subtypes in parkinson's disease. *Brain, 132*(11), 2947–2957.

Shulman, J. M., De Jager, P. L., & Feany, M. B. (2011). Parkinson's disease: Genetics and pathogenesis. *Annual Review of Pathology: Mechanisms of Disease, 6*, 193–222.

Sidtis, D., & Sidtis, J. (2017). Subcortical effects on voice and fluency in dysarthria: Observations from subthalamic nucleus stimulation. *Journal of Alzheimer's Disease & Parkinsonism, 7*(6), 392.

Sidtis, J., Alken, A., Tagliati, M., Alterman, R., & van Lancker Sidtis, D. (2016). Subthalamic stimulation reduces vowel space at the initiation of sustained production: Implications for articulatory motor control in parkinson's disease. *Journal of Parkinson's Disease, 6*(2), 361–370.

Singh, A., Mehrkens, J. H., & Bötzel, K. (2012). Effect of micro lesions of the basal ganglia on ballistic movements in patients with deep brain stimulation. *Journal of the Neurological Sciences, 314*(1-2), 175–177.

Skodda, S. (2015). Die Dysarthrie des Morbus Parkinson: Klinische Präsentation, pathophysiologische und diagnostische Aspekte. *Sprache · Stimme · Gehör, 39*(04), 182–186.

Skodda, S., Grönheit, W., & Schlegel, U. (2011). Intonation and speech rate in parkinson's disease: General and dynamic aspects and responsiveness to levodopa admission. *Journal of Voice, 25*(4), e199–e205.

Skodda, S., Grönheit, W., & Schlegel, U. (2012). Impairment of vowel articulation as a possible marker of disease progression in parkinson's disease. *PLOS ONE*, 7(2), e32132.

Skodda, S., Grönheit, W., Schlegel, U., Südmeyer, M., Schnitzler, A., & Wojtecki, L. (2014). Effect of subthalamic stimulation on voice and speech in parkinson's disease: for the better or worse? *Frontiers in Neurology*, 4, 218.

Skodda, S., & Schlegel, U. (2008). Speech rate and rhythm in parkinson's disease. *Movement Disorders*, 23(7), 985–992.

Skodda, S., Visser, W., & Schlegel, U. (2010). Short-and long-term dopaminergic effects on dysarthria in early parkinson's disease. *Journal of Neural Transmission*, 117(2), 197–205.

Skodda, S., Visser, W., & Schlegel, U. (2011). Vowel articulation in parkinson's disease. *Journal of Voice*, 25(4), 467–472.

Skorvanek, M., Feketeova, E., Kurtis, M. M., Rusz, J., & Sonka, K. (2018). Accuracy of rating scales and clinical measures for screening of rapid eye movement sleep behavior disorder and for predicting conversion to parkinson's disease and other synucleinopathies. *Frontiers in Neurology*, 9, 376.

Spencer, K. A., Morgan, K. W., & Blond, E. (2009). Dopaminergic medication effects on the speech of individuals with parkinson's disease. *Journal of Medical Speech-Language Pathology*, 17(3), 125–145.

Spencer, K. A., & Rogers, M. A. (2005). Speech motor programming in hypokinetic and ataxic dysarthria. *Brain and Language*, 94(3), 347–366.

Sridharan, D., Prashanth, P., & Chakravarthy, V. (2006). The role of the basal ganglia in exploration in a neural model based on reinforcement learning. *International Journal of Neural Systems*, 16(02), 111–124.

Steffman, J. (2021). Contextual prominence in vowel perception: Testing listener sensitivity to sonority expansion and hyperarticulation. *JASA Express Letters*, 1(4), 045203.

Stevens, K. N. (2000). *Acoustic Phonetics* (Vol. 30). MIT press.

Stipancic, K. L., Palmer, K. M., Rowe, H. P., Yunusova, Y., Berry, J. D., & Green, J. R. (2021). "You Say Severe, I Say Mild": Toward an Empirical

Classification of Dysarthria Severity. *Journal of Speech, Language, and Hearing Research*, 64(12), 4718–4735.

Stipancic, K. L., Tjaden, K., & Wilding, G. (2016). Comparison of intelligibility measures for adults with parkinson's disease, adults with multiple sclerosis, and healthy controls. *Journal of Speech, Language, and Hearing Research*, 59(2), 230–238.

Stirpe, P., Hoffman, M., Badiali, D., & Colosimo, C. (2016). Constipation: An emerging risk factor for parkinson's disease? *European Journal of Neurology*, 23(11), 1606–1613.

Svensson, E., Henderson, V. W., Borghammer, P., Horváth-Puhó, E., & Sørensen, H. T. (2016). Constipation and risk of parkinson's disease: A danish population-based cohort study. *Parkinsonism & Related Disorders*, 28, 18–22.

Swets, B., Desmet, T., Hambrick, D. Z., & Ferreira, F. (2007). The role of working memory in syntactic ambiguity resolution: A psychometric approach. *Journal of Experimental Psychology: General*, 136(1), 64–81.

Swets, B., Jacovina, M. E., & Gerrig, R. J. (2013). Effects of conversational pressures on speech planning. *Discourse Processes*, 50(1), 23–51.

Tanaka, Y., Tsuboi, T., Watanabe, H., Kajita, Y., Fujimoto, Y., Ohdake, R., ... Sobue, G. (2015). Voice features of parkinson's disease patients with subthalamic nucleus deep brain stimulation. *Journal of Neurology*, 262(5), 1173–1181.

Tanaka, Y., Tsuboi, T., Watanabe, H., Kajita, Y., Nakatsubo, D., Fujimoto, Y., ... Sobue, G. (2016). Articulation features of parkinson's disease patients with subthalamic nucleus deep brain stimulation. *Journal of Parkinson's Disease*, 6(4), 811–819.

Tanaka, Y., Tsuboi, T., Watanabe, H., Torii, J., Nakatsubo, D., Maesawa, S., ... Katsuno, M. (2021). Instability of speech in parkinson disease patients with subthalamic nucleus deep brain stimulation. *Parkinsonism & Related Disorders*, 93, 8–11.

Tandberg, E., Larsen, J. P., Aarsland, D., Laake, K., & Cummings, J. L. (1997). Risk factors for depression in parkinson disease. *Archives of Neurology*, 54(5), 625–630.

Thies, T., Hermes, A., & Mücke, D. (2022). Compensation in time and space: Prominence marking in aging and disease. *Languages*, 7(1), 21.

Thies, T., Mücke, D., Dano, R., & Barbe, M. T. (2021). Levodopa-based changes on vocalic speech movements during prosodic prominence marking. *Brain Sciences*, *11*(5), 594.

Thies, T., Mücke, D., Lowit, A., Kalbe, E., Steffen, J., & Barbe, M. T. (2020). Prominence marking in parkinsonian speech and its correlation with motor performance and cognitive abilities. *Neuropsychologia*, *137*, 107306.

Thompson, A. R. (2018). *Articulatory kinematics during stop closure in speakers with parkinson's disease* (Master's thesis). Louisiana State University, Communication Sciences and Disorders.

Tjaden, K., Lam, J., & Wilding, G. (2013). Vowel acoustics in parkinson's disease and multiple sclerosis: Comparison of clear, loud, and slow speaking conditions. *Journal of Speech, Language, and Hearing Research*, *56*(5), 1485 – 1502.

Tjaden, K., & Martel-Sauvageau, V. (2017). Consonant acoustics in parkinson's disease and multiple sclerosis: Comparison of clear and loud speaking conditions. *American Journal of Speech-Language Pathology*, *26*(2S), 569–582.

Tjaden, K., Sussman, J. E., & Wilding, G. E. (2014). Impact of clear, loud, and slow speech on scaled intelligibility and speech severity in parkinson's disease and multiple sclerosis. *Journal of Speech, Language, and Hearing Research*, *57*(3), 779–792.

Tomlinson, C. L., Stowe, R., Patel, S., Rick, C., Gray, R., & Clarke, C. E. (2010). Systematic review of levodopa dose equivalency reporting in parkinson's disease. *Movement Disorders*, *25*(15), 2649–2653.

Tripoliti, E., Dowsey-Limousin, P., Tisch, S., Borrell, E., & Hariz, M. I. (2006). Speech in parkinson's disease following subthalamic nucleus deep brain stimulation: preliminary results. *Journal of Medical Speech-Language Pathology*, *14*(4), 309–316.

Tripoliti, E., Zrinzo, L., Martinez-Torres, I., Frost, E., Pinto, S., Foltynie, T., ... Limousin, P. (2011). Effects of subthalamic stimulation on speech of consecutive patients with parkinson disease. *Neurology*, *76*(1), 80–86.

Tsao, Y.-C., Weismer, G., & Iqbal, K. (2006). Interspeaker variation in habitual speaking rate: Additional evidence. *Journal of Speech, Language, and Hearing Research*, 40(4), 858–866.

Tsuboi, T., Watanabe, H., Tanaka, Y., Ohdake, R., Yoneyama, N., Hara, K., ... Sobue, G. (2015). Distinct phenotypes of speech and voice disorders in parkinson's disease after subthalamic nucleus deep brain stimulation. *Journal of Neurology, Neurosurgery & Psychiatry*, 86(8), 856–864.

Turkmani, A., Hilton, A., Jackson, P. J., & Edge, J. (2007). Visual analysis of lip coarticulation in vcv utterances. In *Proceedings of 8th Annual Conference of the International Speech Communication Association* (pp. 1281–1284).

Tykalová, T., Rusz, J., Cmejla, R., Růžička, H., & Ruzicka, E. (2014). Acoustic investigation of stress patterns in parkinson's disease. *Journal of Voice*, 28(1), 129.E1–129.E8.

Tykalová, T., Rusz, J., Švihlík, J., Bancone, S., Spezia, A., & Pellecchia, M. T. (2020). Speech disorder and vocal tremor in postural instability/gait difficulty and tremor dominant subtypes of parkinson's disease. *Journal of Neural Transmission*, 127(9), 1295–1304.

Tykocki, T., Nauman, P., Koziara, H., & Mandat, T. (2013). Microlesion effect as a predictor of the effectiveness of subthalamic deep brain stimulation for parkinson's disease. *Stereotactic and Functional Neurosurgery*, 91(1), 12–17.

Tysnes, O.-B., & Storstein, A. (2017). Epidemiology of parkinson's disease. *Journal of Neural Transmission*, 124(8), 901–905.

Van Den Eeden, S. K., Tanner, C. M., Bernstein, A. L., Fross, R. D., Leimpeter, A., Bloch, D. A., & Nelson, L. M. (2003). Incidence of Parkinson's disease: Variation by Age, Gender, and Race/Ethnicity. *American Journal of Epidemiology*, 157(11), 1015–1022.

van Hartevelt, T. J., Cabral, J., Deco, G., Møller, A., Green, A. L., Aziz, T. Z., & Kringelbach, M. L. (2014). Neural plasticity in human brain connectivity: The effects of long term deep brain stimulation of the subthalamic nucleus in parkinson's disease. *PLOS ONE*, 9(1), e86496.

van Heuven, V. J., & Sluijter, A. M. (1996). Notes on the phonetics of word prosody. In R. Goedemans, H. Hulst, & E. Visch (Eds.), *Stress Patterns of the World, Part 1: Background* (pp. 233–269). Holland Academic Graphics.

van Lancker Sidtis, D., Rogers, T., Godier, V., Tagliati, M., & Sidtis, J. (2010). Voice and fluency changes as a function of speech task and deep brain stimulation. *Journal of Speech, Language, and Hearing Research*, 53(5), 1167–1177.

Vitek, J. L. (2002). Deep brain stimulation for parkinson's disease. *Stereotactic and Functional Neurosurgery*, 78(3-4), 119–131.

Walsh, B., & Smith, A. (2012). Basic parameters of articulatory movements and acoustics in individuals with parkinson's disease. *Movement Disorders*, 27(7), 843–850.

Wang, E., Metman, L. V., Bakay, R., Arzbaecher, J., Bernard, B., & Corcos, D. (2006). Hemisphere-specific effects of subthalamic nucleus deep brain stimulation on speaking rate and articulatory accuracy of syllable repetitions in parkinson's disease. *Journal of Medical Speech-Language Pathology*, 14(4), 323.

Wang, Y., Li, P., Gong, F., Gao, Y., Xu, Y. Y., & Wang, W. (2017). Micro lesion effect of the globus pallidus internus with deep brain stimulation in parkinson's disease patients. *Acta Neurochirurgica*, 159(9), 1727–1731.

Weicker, H., Kinscherf, R., Diserens, K., Deigner, H.-P., & Strüder, H. (2001). Physiology and pathophysiology of basalganglia: Impact on motor system function. *European Journal of Sport Science*, 1(2), 1–46.

Weintraub, D., Koester, J., Potenza, M. N., Siderowf, A. D., Stacy, M., Voon, V., ... Lang, A. E. (2010). Impulse control disorders in parkinson disease: A cross-sectional study of 3090 patients. *Archives of Neurology*, 67(5), 589–595.

Weir-Mayta, P., Spencer, K. A., Eadie, T. L., Yorkston, K., Savaglio, S., & Woollcott, C. (2017). Internally versus externally cued speech in parkinson's disease and cerebellar disease. *American Journal of Speech-Language Pathology*, 26(2S), 583–595.

Weismer, G., Jeng, J.-Y., Laures, J. S., Kent, R. D., & Kent, J. F. (2001). Acoustic and intelligibility characteristics of sentence production in neurogenic speech disorders. *Folia Phoniatrica et Logopaedica*, 53(1), 1–18.

Weismer, G., Yunusova, Y., & Bunton, K. (2012). Measures to evaluate the effects of dbs on speech production. *Journal of Neurolinguistics*, 25(2), 74–94.

Weismer, G., Yunusova, Y., & Westbury, J. R. (2003). Interarticulator coordination in dysarthria. *Journal of Speech, Language, and Hearing Research*, 1247–1261.

Welter, M., Houeto, J., Tezenas du Montcel, S., Mesnage, V., Bonnet, A., Pillon, B., ... Agid, Y. (2002). Clinical predictive factors of subthalamic stimulation in parkinson's disease. *Brain*, 125(3), 575–583.

Whitehill, T. L., & Wong, C. C.-Y. (2006). Contributing factors to listener effort for dysarthric speech. *Journal of Medical Speech-Language Pathology*, 14(4), 335–342.

Whitfield, J., & Goberman, A. (2014). Articulatory–acoustic vowel space: Application to clear speech in individuals with parkinson's disease. *Journal of Communication Disorders*, 51, 19–28.

WHO. (2001). *International Classification of Functioning, Disability and Health: ICF*. World Health Organization.

Winkelmann, R., Harrington, J., & Jänsch, K. (2017). EMU-SDMS: Advanced speech database management and analysis in R. *Computer Speech & Language*, 45, 392–410.

Winkelmann, R., Jaensch, K., Cassidy, S., & Harrington, J. (2021). emuR: Main Package of the EMU Speech Database Management System [Computer software manual]. (R package version 2.3.0)

Wirsching, I., Buttmann, M., Odorfer, T., Volkmann, J., Classen, J., & Zeller, D. (2018). Altered motor plasticity in an acute relapse of multiple sclerosis. *European Journal of Neuroscience*, 47(3), 251–257.

Witt, K., Granert, O., Daniels, C., Volkmann, J., Falk, D., van Eimeren, T., & Deuschl, G. (2013). Relation of lead trajectory and electrode position to neuropsychological outcomes of subthalamic neurostimulation in parkinson's disease: results from a randomized trial. *Brain*, 136(7), 2109–2119.

Wong, M. N., Murdoch, B. E., & Whelan, B.-M. (2011). Lingual kinematics in dysarthric and nondysarthric speakers with parkinson's disease. *Parkinson's Disease*, 352838.

Xie, Y., Zhang, Y., Zheng, Z., Liu, A., Wang, X., Zhuang, P., ... Wang, X. (2011). Changes in speech characters of patients with parkinson's disease after bilateral subthalamic nucleus stimulation. *Journal of Voice*, 25(6), 751–758.

Yorkston, K. M., Beukelman, D. R., & Bell, K. R. (1988). *Clinical Management of Dysarthric Speakers*. Little Brown.

Yorkston, K. M., Beukelman, D. R., Strand, E. A., & Hakel, M. (1999). *Management of Motor Speech Disorders in Children and Adults* (Vol. 404). Pro Ed: Austin, Texas.

Yunusova, Y., Weismer, G., Westbury, J. R., & Lindstrom, M. J. (2008). Articulatory movements during vowels in speakers with dysarthria and healthy controls. *Journal of Speech, Language, and Hearing Research*, 51(3), 596 – 611.

Zhang, J., Zhang, K., Ma, Y., Hu, W., Yang, A., Chu, J., ... Wang, Z. (2006). Follow-up of bilateral subthalamic deep brain stimulation for parkinson's disease. In J. W. Chang, Y. Katayama, & T. Yamamoto (Eds.), *Advances in Functional and Reparative Neurosurgery* (pp. 43–47). Springer.

Zhou, L., Zhu, L., & Liu, J. (2018). From rapid eye movement sleep behavior disorder to parkinson's disease: Possible predictive markers of conversion. *ACS Chemical Neuroscience*, 10(2), 824–827.

Ziegler, W. (2002). Task-related factors in oral motor control: Speech and oral diadochokinesis in dysarthria and apraxia of speech. *Brain and Language*, 80(3), 556–575.

Ziegler, W. (2017). Physiologie und zentralnervöse Organisation des Sprechens und deren Veränderung unter Morbus Parkinson. In A. Nebel & G. Deuschl (Eds.), *Dysarthrie und Dysphagie bei Morbus Parkinson* (2nd ed., pp. 76–91). Georg Thieme Verlag.

Ziegler, W., & Vogel, M. (2010). *Dysarthrie: verstehen-untersuchen-behandeln*. Georg Thieme Verlag.

Speech Production and Perception
Edited by Susanne Fuchs and Pascal Perrier

Vol. 1   Susanne Fuchs / Melanie Weirich / Daniel Pape / Pascal Perrier (eds.): Speech Planning and Dynamics. 2012.

Vol. 2   Anne Hermes: Articulatory Coordination and Syllable Structure in Italian. 2013.

Vol. 3   Susanne Fuchs / Daniel Pape / Caterina Petrone / Pascal Perrier (eds.): Individual Differences in Speech Production and Perception. 2015.

Vol. 4   Louis-Jean Boë / Joël Fagot / Pascal Perrier / Jean-Luc Schwartz (eds.): Origins of Human Language: Continuities and Discontinuities with Nonhuman Primates. 2017.

Vol. 5   Jessica Di Napoli: The Phonetics and Phonology of Glottalization in Italian. 2018.

Vol. 6   Susanne Fuchs / Joanne Cleland / Amélie Rochet-Capellan (eds.): Speech production and perception: Learning and memory. 2019.

Vol. 7   Tabea Thies: Tongue Body Kinematics in Parkinson's Disease. Effects of Levodopa and Deep Brain Stimulation. 2023.

www.peterlang.com

www.ingramcontent.com/pod-product-compliance
Ingram Content Group UK Ltd.
Pitfield, Milton Keynes, MK11 3LW, UK
UKHW021822140426
5217IPUK00004B/46